21 THINGS
YOU NEED TO KNOW ABOUT
DIABETES

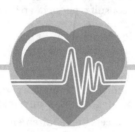

and

YOUR HEART

Jill Weisenberger, MS, RDN, CDE, FAND

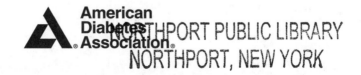

American
Diabetes
Association®

Director, Book Publishing, Abe Ogden; Managing Editor, Greg Guthrie; Acquisitions Editor, Victor Van Beuren; Editor, Kim Douglass Marin; Production Manager, Melissa Sprott; Composition, ADA; Cover Design, Jody Billert; Printer, United Graphics.

Printed in the United States of America
1 3 5 7 9 10 8 6 4 2

The suggestions and information contained in this publication are generally consistent with the *Clinical Practice Recommendations* and other policies of the American Diabetes Association, but they do not represent the policy or position of the Association or any of its boards or committees. Reasonable steps have been taken to ensure the accuracy of the information presented. However, the American Diabetes Association cannot ensure the safety or efficacy of any product or service described in this publication. Individuals are advised to consult a physician or other appropriate health care professional before undertaking any diet or exercise program or taking any medication referred to in this publication. Professionals must use and apply their own professional judgment, experience, and training and should not rely solely on the information contained in this publication before prescribing any diet, exercise, or medication. The American Diabetes Association—its officers, directors, employees, volunteers, and members—assumes no responsibility or liability for personal or other injury, loss, or damage that may result from the suggestions or information in this publication.

♾ The paper in this publication meets the requirements of the ANSI Standard Z39.48-1992 (permanence of paper).

ADA titles may be purchased for business or promotional use or for special sales. To purchase more than 50 copies of this book at a discount, or for custom editions of this book with your logo, contact the American Diabetes Association at the address below or at booksales@diabetes.org.

American Diabetes Association
1701 North Beauregard Street
Alexandria, Virginia 22311

DOI: 10.2337/9781580405409

Library of Congress Cataloging-in-Publication Data
Weisenberger, Jill.
 21 things you need to know about diabetes and your heart / Jill Weisenberger, MS, RDN, CDE, FAND.
     pages cm
Summary: «This book illustrates how heart disease is a serious health threat, especially for people with diabetes. In fact, it is responsible for one in four deaths in the United States and is the leading cause of death among both men and women. Unfortunately, having diabetes at least doubles your risk of heart trouble. The good news is that there is a lot we can do to treat it and to protect ourselves from developing this life-threatening disease.»-- Provided by publisher.
 Includes bibliographical references and index.
 ISBN 978-1-58040-540-9 (paperback)
1. Heart--Diseases. 2. Diabetes--Complications. I. Title. II. Title: Twenty one things you need to know about diabetes and your heart.
 RC682.W423 2014
 641.5'6311--dc23
                            2014025791

Table of Contents

Foreword

I am certain you are aware of heart disease, and you probably know it is the number one cause of death in the United States. That means heart disease will probably kill you. It's a sobering thought. In fact, we are in the middle of an epidemic of heart disease, and just about everyone is affected.

However, did you know that heart disease is preventable? It really is. Did you know that it is reversible if you already have it? How do we know this? First, there are whole populations of people in this world who rarely are affected by heart disease. For example, the Tarahumara Native Americans living in Mexico rarely get heart disease, that is until they move to the United States and assume our way of living.

Most animals rarely get heart disease, unless they are fed a high-fat diet. People who eat certain diets (such as the Mediterranean diet in Europe) have a low incidence of heart disease compared to people who eat a Westernized diet. Randomized, controlled clinical trials using medications that reduce the circulating blood level of cholesterol have demonstrated a marked reduction in heart disease. And finally, direct heart artery observation studies using intravascular ultrasound (a picture of an artery using sound waves) have convincingly shown a reversal of atherosclerosis when blood cholesterol is significantly reduced. So we know some things work.

How do *you* stop atherosclerosis from building up in your arteries and eventually causing a heart attack? The good news is that the answer is not "rocket science." The bad news is that you will have to do a little homework. In essence, you will have to get smart about heart disease.

And that is where this excellent book comes in. Jill Weisenberger has created a great reference, full of good ideas and suggestions. It gives examples of people like you who want to live healthy and smart. It will lead you in the right direction, and it may save your life. Just don't read it once and think you know all you need to know. You won't. You'll need to read it again and again.

Here are my suggestions: Underline the key points in the book that you want to remember. Dog-ear the pages that are especially helpful. Bookmark the chapters that you need to read again. In other words, use it to prevent or reverse heart disease in you. Then, as an act of kindness, buy your spouse, partner, or neighbor a copy, because you sure don't want to give him/her yours. Not on your life!

—David S. Schade, MD
  Distinguished and Regents' Professor of Medicine;
  Chief, Division of Endocrinology,
  University of New Mexico Health Sciences Center,
  Albuquerque, NM

Acknowledgments

Many thanks to the American Diabetes Association for allowing me this opportunity to teach and encourage people with diabetes to care for their hearts. I appreciate the hard work that goes into polishing a book idea, and designing, illustrating, and editing the text. I appreciate also the reviewers for their time, expertise, and wise comments. Thank you to all who have worked on this project.

It is my patients who inspired me to write on this topic. Thank you for sharing your stories and struggles.

My family—including my four-legged family members—keeps me sane and entertained, no matter what I'm working on. Thank you for being you.

What Is Heart Disease?

There is no denying that heart disease is a serious health threat, especially for people with diabetes. In fact, it is responsible for one in four deaths in the United States and is the leading cause of death among both men and women. Unfortunately, having diabetes at least doubles your risk of heart trouble. The good news, as you will see in later chapters, is that there is a lot we can do to treat and protect ourselves from developing this life-threatening heart disease. In the first few chapters, however, we discuss the disease process.

Heart disease, or cardiovascular disease (CVD), is the catchall term to describe diseases of the heart or the blood vessels. The most common form of heart disease is coronary artery disease (CAD), which occurs when the inner walls of the arteries that carry blood to the heart muscle become streaked or lined with plaque. Plaque is a sticky material made of fat, cholesterol, calcium, and other substances from your blood.

The troublesome buildup of plaque is called atherosclerosis, which comes from the Greek roots meaning "hardening" and "gruel." Atherosclerosis can limit blood flow to the heart (and tissues in other parts of the body), leaving the heart muscle without the adequate oxygen and nutrients it needs to function properly. If the plaque ruptures, a blood clot will form inside the artery. If the clot is large enough, it can partially or completely block the flow of blood to the heart.

Atherosclerosis can start at a young age and progress over decades. It can smolder throughout adulthood, causing no noticeable symptoms for many years. It's easy to take the health of your heart and blood vessels for granted when you feel fine and can't see through your skin at the structure and function of your organs. Having and dealing with diabetes already takes up energy and time and gives you lots to tend to—so much, in fact, that it may seem that diabetes is like a full-time job. Having to focus on the health of your heart is an extra burden. Indeed, you may need additional medical tests and medications. But fortunately, many of the things you already do to tend to your diabetes, including eating a healthy diet, exercising, and controlling your blood glucose, do double duty and protect your heart, too. Don't take your heart for granted. A healthy heart will enable you to enjoy an active life now and in all the years to come.

Symptoms of Coronary Artery Disease

While there may be no symptoms at all, you may experience any of the following:

> Angina: a squeezing pain or pressing feeling in your chest that may come and go. It may also feel like indigestion.

> Shortness of breath, especially during physical activity

> Arrhythmia: irregular heart beating. It may feel as if your heart is beating too quickly or skipping beats.

> Heart attack (see chapter 3)

The Mighty Endothelial Cells

To understand how atherosclerosis occurs, imagine a healthy blood vessel as a clean, hollow tube through which blood flows easily. It's lined with a thin layer of specialized cells called the endothelium. For such a thin layer of protection, these endothelial cells do mighty work and perform numerous critical functions to maintain healthy blood vessels throughout the body. The endothelium acts as a barrier that contains blood within the lumen (the canal of the blood vessels), limits the passage of large compounds from the blood into the deeper layers of the blood vessel walls, and secretes substances that keep cells and other compounds in the bloodstream from sticking to it. The endothelial cells also secrete nitric oxide (NO), a chemical that dilates or relaxes blood vessels. When this lining becomes damaged, it sets the stage for atherosclerosis. Fatty substances pass into the vessel wall, inflammatory compounds are released, the blood vessel doesn't relax as well, and there is less resistance to the formation of a dangerous blood clot.

The Formation of Atherosclerosis

Fatty streaks are the first visible signs of atherosclerosis, and they appear as a yellow discoloration within the artery wall. These fatty streaks likely form when high blood pressure, diabetes, chemicals from tobacco smoke, or other toxic substances assault the endothelium. Low-density lipoprotein, also called LDL (bad) cholesterol, passes beneath the damaged endothelial lining through the intima, the first layer of the arterial wall. If you have elevated LDL cholesterol, the LDL particles can infiltrate the intima at a faster rate. Within the intima, LDL cholesterol becomes modified or oxidized. Having high blood glucose may increase LDL modification.

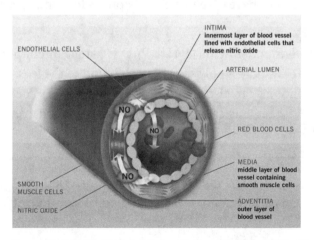

Source: National Institutes on Aging, National Institutes of Health

Now that the LDL cholesterol has made its way into the blood vessel wall and has become chemically altered, the inflammatory process is activated, and metabolic mayhem ensues. Immune cells are summoned, and in an attempt to destroy the fatty substance, the immune cells swallow it. They then become foam cells, so called because of their foamy, fatty appearance. Foam cells die and stimulate the inflammatory process even more. It becomes a cycle of damage, inflammation, and more damage and inflammation. The progression of plaque involves the middle layer of the blood vessel wall as well. Smooth muscle cells from the media migrate into the intima, where they alter the structure and integrity further. By removing or reducing the source of damage to the endothelium—high blood pressure, elevated cholesterol, cigarette smoke, and others—we can slow the progression of atherosclerosis.

Atherosclerosis in Other Blood Vessels

Plaque can build up in any artery of the body, including arteries in the brain, arms, legs, and kidneys.

➤ *Carotid artery disease.* Atherosclerosis of the arteries on each side of the neck, the carotid arteries, can hinder blood flow to the brain and cause a stroke. The risk of having an ischemic stroke—the type caused by a blocked blood vessel—is three times as great if you have had diabetes for 10 years or more compared to people your age who do not have diabetes. See chapter 3 for symptoms of a stroke.

➤ *Peripheral arterial disease (PAD).* PAD is plaque buildup in the major arteries that supply oxygen-rich blood to the legs. Though less common, it can also affect the arms and pelvis. Blocked blood flow to these regions can cause numbness, pain, and even infections. Peripheral vascular disease (PVD) is another way to describe the same thing.

➤ *Renal artery disease.* Atherosclerosis in the arteries leading to the kidneys can cause high blood pressure and a slow loss of kidney function.

Coronary Artery Disease = Coronary Heart Disease

Many experts declare that there is a difference between coronary artery disease (CAD) and coronary heart disease (CHD). They say: CAD starts first and leads to CHD. But in this book, the terms are used interchangeably.

Is Inflammation to Blame?

Low-grade chronic inflammation is associated with heart disease. Inflammation can be both good and bad. It's a good thing if you cut your hand, for example. The body launches an attack with white blood cells. You will notice redness and swelling as these immune cells come together at the site of injury to rid your body of bacteria or other foreign invaders. This is an acute inflammatory response that ends fairly quickly.

The damage to an artery is ongoing, however. The body sees plaque as a foreign invader and summons immune cells to the artery wall. The inflammatory response continues, long term, and can lead to further damage.

Congestive Heart Failure

Coronary artery disease may eventually lead to congestive heart failure (CHF), often simply referred to as heart failure. High blood pressure and diabetes also increase a person's risk of developing CHF. Though it is very serious, heart failure is not the death sentence it may sound like. CHF is a condition in which the heart cannot pump enough blood to meet the body's needs. Sometimes the heart does not fill with enough blood. Other times, the heart lacks the force to pump the blood to the rest of the body. Symptoms of CHF include:

> shortness of breath (difficulty breathing during exercise and sometimes at rest). This is caused by fluid leaking into the lungs when the heart does not pump properly.

> persistent coughing or wheezing (also caused by fluid in the lungs)

> edema (swelling in the ankles, feet, legs, or abdomen). This is caused by fluid building up in the tissues instead of making its way back to the heart. It may cause weight gain.

> fatigue

Health-care professionals typically classify patients with CHF according to their symptoms. Class I identifies patients with only mild symptoms. Class IV is the classification designated to patients with the most severe symptoms. These individuals experience discomfort with any level of physical activity.

Many of the lifestyle strategies described later in this book for the treatment and prevention of coronary artery disease and stroke are appropriate for the treatment of CHF as well. However, if you have CHF, your health-care provider may prescribe additional dietary measures such as changing your food and beverage intake.

The Sad Facts About Heart Disease

➤ At least 26.5 million Americans adults have diagnosed heart disease.
➤ About 600,000 people in the United States die of heart disease every year. Heart disease is the leading cause of death among Americans.
➤ Coronary artery disease is responsible for 385,000 deaths each year, more than any other form of heart disease.
➤ Coronary artery disease costs the United States $108.9 billion annually in health-care services, medications, and lost productivity.
➤ Each year about 715,000 Americans suffer a heart attack. For 525,000 of them, it's their first heart attack.

Source: Centers for Disease Control and Prevention

The Diabetes–Heart Disease Connection

When we talk about diabetes, we usually put most of the emphasis on blood sugar or blood glucose. That's not surprising since diabetes is defined by high blood glucose. While controlling and monitoring blood glucose is critical, we also need to pay special attention to those aspects of our health that are not so immediate, including the health of the heart, blood vessels, and other organ systems.

Unfortunately, people with diabetes have a high risk for heart disease. Blood vessel damage throughout the body occurs more frequently, at an earlier age, and with greater severity in people with diabetes compared to those without diabetes. Diabetes is an independent risk factor for cardiovascular disease, doubling or tripling the risk in men and even more in women. Though these statistics sound very scary, good lifestyle habits help put you in control of your health. Furthermore, medical management of risk factors and other health problems greatly improves your chances of leading a full life without heart disease. The key is to consistently make smart food, exercise, and other lifestyle choices and to discuss medical management with your health-care team. Many of the following chapters will guide you in doing these things.

Diabetes as a Risk Factor

There are many possible ways that diabetes raises your risk of heart disease. As you saw in chapter 1, atherosclerosis is the hallmark of coronary artery disease. Having elevated blood glucose may cause endothelial dysfunction, damage blood vessels, and modify LDL cholesterol, which spur the process of atherosclerosis. Additionally, people with diabetes tend to have problems with blood vessel dilation and a greater likelihood of forming blood clots that can obstruct blood flow.

Type 2 diabetes is characterized by insulin resistance, which is the inability of some of the body's cells to properly use insulin. After drinking a cup of milk, eating an apple, or consuming any other carbohydrate-rich food, the blood receives a healthy dose of glucose. The pancreas then sends out insulin to help usher excess glucose out of the blood and into the muscle and fat cells. There, glucose is used for energy or stored for later use. When fat and muscle cells first become resistant to insulin's action, the pancreas cranks out more and more insulin to do the job, much as a baby's cries become louder and louder when the mother fails to respond.

In the earlier stages of insulin resistance, blood glucose levels normalize without any sign that something is awry. Blood glucose levels may first rise to the level of prediabetes and then to the level of diabetes (see box below), and all the while, insulin levels in the blood are higher than normal. These elevated insulin levels may occur for years before a diagnosis of type 2 diabetes.

Researchers now believe that this resistance to insulin and elevated insulin levels play an important role in the development of coronary artery disease even in people who do not have diabetes. This is because insulin has many roles in the body unrelated to blood glucose. Insulin resistance also affects blood pressure, blood cholesterol and triglyceride levels, blood clotting, and even more risk factors for heart disease. You will learn more about these risk factors in chapter 4.

Blood Glucose Levels to Diagnose Diabetes and Prediabetes

Test	Prediabetes	Diabetes
Fasting plasma glucose	100–125 mg/dl	≥126 mg/dl
2-hour oral glucose tolerance test (OGTT)	140–199 mg/dl	≥200 mg/dl
Random plasma glucose in a person with symptoms of diabetes, such as frequent urination and excessive thirst	—	≥200 mg/dl
A1C	5.7–6.4%	≥6.5%

Source: American Diabetes Association Clinical Practice Recommendations (2014)

Symptoms of a Heart Attack

Maggie, aged 54 years, was fighting nausea, and she couldn't stop sweating. She came up with a bunch of excuses for feeling poorly, but having a heart attack wasn't one of them. Maybe she was coming down with the flu, and it was an especially hot day, too. She also wondered if she had food poisoning from her lunch at the new restaurant earlier in the day. It was a lifesaver that Maggie's coworker knew the signs of a heart attack and convinced Maggie to seek medical help.

On Monday morning, Jack, aged 39 years, woke up with pain in the center of his chest as well as in his left arm, his back, and neck. He brushed it off as soreness from doing too much yard work over the weekend. Later in the morning, he still had no appetite for breakfast and felt just a bit short of breath. He felt silly doing it, thinking he was making a big deal out of nothing, but he called 911 anyway. It's a good thing he did, because Jack was having a heart attack.

These stories illustrate several important things:

➤ You don't have to be an old man to have a heart attack.

➤ The signs and symptoms of a heart attack may be very different from movie scenes in which the person having the heart attack grabs his chest, gasps, and collapses.

➤ Seeking immediate help can save your life.

What Is a Heart Attack?

When blood flow to a section of the heart is blocked, that part of the heart muscle is starved for oxygen and nutrients, resulting in ischemia. If damage or death occurs to part of the heart muscle, it is called a heart attack. Cardiac arrest is different; it can be caused by a heart attack or by something else. Cardiac arrest is a malfunction in the heart's electrical system. It results in death when the heart suddenly stops working properly. Cardiac arrest can be reversed with CPR (cardiopulmonary resuscitation) and an AED (automated external defibrillator). Most heart attacks do not lead to cardiac arrest.

A Heart Attack By Any Other Name

Medical professionals toss around a lot of words that mean the same thing. The medical term for a heart attack is myocardial infarction (MI). A coronary thrombosis is the formation of a blood clot in an artery of the heart. Coronary occlusion is an obstruction in a coronary artery. Health professionals may use any of these terms to refer to a heart attack.

Know When to Call 911

Since the signs of a heart attack vary from person to person (and even from first or second heart attack to second or third heart attack), when in doubt, call 911. Don't waste precious time waiting to see if things get worse or searching for the symptoms of a heart attack on the Internet. Here are some of the more common signs:

Chest pain or discomfort. This can range from feeling like an elephant is sitting on your chest to mild or severe squeezing or pain to fullness or discomfort that is similar to indigestion. The pain or discomfort may last several minutes, or it may come and go.

Upper body discomfort. You may experience pain or discomfort in one or both arms, your neck, back, shoulders, jaw, or stomach.

Shortness of breath. You may feel a little out of breath when resting or when doing light physical activity. This can occur even if you do not have chest pain.

The following are less common signs of a heart attack:

> Nausea and vomiting

> Breaking out in a cold sweat

> Feeling unusually tired for no apparent reason

> Sudden dizziness or feeling light-headed

Chest pain or discomfort is the most common sign among both men and women. Women, however, are more likely than men to experience other symptoms. Additionally, diabetic nerve damage or other neuropathy (nerve disorder) may cause symptoms to be milder or even mask the symptoms of a heart attack.

If you think you might be having a heart attack, get to a hospital immediately. It's best to go by ambulance, because emergency medical technicians can start lifesaving treatments or medications.

Is It a Heart Attack or Angina?

Angina is chest pain or discomfort that commonly occurs in people with coronary artery disease when they are physically active. This type of pain usually lasts for only a few minutes and goes away with rest. Chest pain or discomfort that doesn't go away or that feels different from your typical angina discomfort may be a sign that you are having a heart attack. If you're not sure what your chest pain means, call for emergency medical help right away.

Symptoms of a Stroke

Recall that plaque may build up in blood vessels in any part of the body, including the arteries that carry blood to the brain. People with diabetes also have an increased risk for stroke. The American Stroke Association has a "F.A.S.T." method to identify the sudden signs of stroke. If you spot these signs of a stroke, call 911 or your emergency number right away.

F **Face Drooping**: Does one side of the face droop, or is it numb? Ask the person to smile. Is the person's smile uneven?

A **Arm Weakness**: Is one arm weak or numb? Ask the person to raise both arms. Does one arm drift downward?

S **Speech Difficulty**: Is speech slurred? Is the person unable to speak or hard to understand? Ask the person to repeat a simple sentence, like "The sky is blue." Is the sentence repeated correctly?

T **Time to call 911**: If someone shows any of these symptoms, even if the symptoms go away, call 911 and get the person to the hospital immediately. Check the time so you will know when the first symptoms appeared.

Take Action

Talk to a member of your health-care team about the warning signs of a heart attack and a stroke. Ask if you are likely to have unusual symptoms. Commit the warning signs to memory.

The Risk Factors for
Coronary Artery Disease

There are some risk factors, such as age and family history of premature heart disease, which we can't do a thing about. This makes it all the more important to work hard at reducing the risk factors we *can* control. One thing we do know is that the more risk factors you have, the greater your overall risk. Happily, even if you are at high risk right now, there are things you can do to lower your risk.

Risk Factors You Can't Control

There are three major risk factors that you cannot control:

Age. With each birthday, your risk for heart disease increases. According to the American Heart Association, 82% of people who die from coronary artery disease are aged 65 years or older.

Gender. In the general population, men have a greater risk for coronary artery disease, but as women age, their risk approaches that of men. However, a woman with diabetes loses the protection of her gender: She has the same risk for coronary artery disease as a man of the same age with diabetes.

Family history and genetics. You are at greater risk for heart disease if your parents or siblings developed it. Heart disease risk is also elevated among African-Americans, Mexican-Americans, American Indians, native Hawaiians, and some Asian-Americans.

Risk Factors You Can Control

You can do a lot to keep your heart in tip-top shape. A heart-healthy lifestyle and medications, if prescribed, can lower your risk for coronary artery disease. Below are several risk factors for heart disease over which you have some level of control. Several of the following risk factors are discussed in greater detail in other chapters.

Blood pressure. Blood pressure is the force of blood pushing against blood vessel walls. When it is high, the force on the arteries is too great and can cause tiny tears in the artery wall. As you saw in chapter 1, this sets the stage for atherosclerosis. High blood pressure, or hypertension, is often called the silent killer because it has no symptoms. Yet it is the leading cause of stroke and can also lead to heart attack and heart failure, kidney damage, vision loss, erectile dysfunction, and other health problems. You will learn more about high blood pressure in chapters 7 and 8.

Cholesterol. Cholesterol is a waxy substance that is found in the bodies of all animals. Some comes from the foods we eat, but most of the cholesterol is made within our own bodies. Cholesterol is an important part of our cell membranes, and it's used to make some hormones and vitamin D. However, if you have too much cholesterol in the blood, especially LDL cholesterol, you are at increased risk for coronary artery disease. Remember from chapter 1 that LDL cholesterol enters the blood vessel wall beneath the endothelium. Once it has made its way into the intima, it becomes chemically modified, damaging the artery wall further and perpetuating the development of atherosclerosis. Chapters 9 and 10 are dedicated to a thorough discussion of cholesterol.

Triglycerides. Triglycerides are the most common type of fat in your body and in your food. They are not a type of cholesterol, but are frequently measured the same time your blood cholesterol is measured. According to the American Heart Association, a high triglyceride level, combined with an abnormal cholesterol level, speeds up atherosclerosis. Triglycerides are discussed again in chapter 9.

Diabetes. Diabetes is a major risk factor for cardiovascular disease. Diabetes may increase the risk of heart disease because of elevated blood glucose as well as the influences of insulin resistance on blood pressure, cholesterol, triglycerides, blood clotting, endothelial function, inflammation, and more. The link between diabetes and heart disease was discussed in greater detail in chapter 2.

Metabolic syndrome. Metabolic syndrome is not really *a* risk factor. Rather it is a cluster or a group of risk factors: high blood pressure, abnormal cholesterol, elevated triglycerides, high fasting blood glucose, and excess fat around the abdomen. Having three or more of these abnormalities means that you have metabolic syndrome, which puts you at increased risk for both type 2 diabetes and cardiovascular disease. Several organizations have criteria for diagnosing metabolic syndrome. Below is one common set of criteria.

Clinical Criteria for the Diagnosis of the Metabolic Syndrome

Abdominal obesity	Waist circumference
—Men	>40 inches
—Women	>35 inches
Triglycerides	>150 mg/dl
High-density lipoprotein (HDL) cholesterol	
—Men	<40 mg/dl
—Women	<50 mg/dl
Blood pressure	>130/>85 mmHg
Fasting blood glucose	>110 mg/dl

Source: U.S. Expert Panel on Detection, Evaluation, and Treatment of High Blood Cholesterol in Adults (Adult Treatment Panel III)

Measuring Your Waist

To measure your waist properly, place the tape measure just above the tip of your hipbone. The tape measure should be snug without pinching your skin. Exhale before reading the tape measure.

Overweight and obesity. Nearly 70% of American adults are either overweight or obese. This poses many serious health threats. Body fat is not inert. Excess body fat does more than just sit on our bodies making our clothes feel tight or causing us to feel self-conscious. Fat tissue is actually busy at work sending out dozens of chemicals that set the stage for heart disease, type 2 diabetes, and many other chronic diseases. Carrying excess fat around the middle seems to be even more dangerous than excess fat at the hips, thighs, and other parts of the body.

Most people can simply look in the mirror to see if they are overweight. Even so, it helps to have an objective measure to assess an individual's level of overweight or obesity. Health-care providers and researchers often use the Body Mass Index (BMI) as a screening tool to identify possible weight problems. You can visit the website of the American Diabetes Association (ADA) to calculate your BMI (diabetes. org/food-and-fitness/weight-loss/assess-your-lifestyle/bmi-tool.html), use the chart on the website of the National Heart, Lung, and Blood Institute (NHLBI) (nhlbi.nih.gov/guidelines/obesity/bmi_tbl.htm), or use the following formula. (Children and teens, however, have a separate BMI calculator, which can be found at apps.nccd.cdc.gov/dnpabmi/.)

BMI: Weight (in pounds) / [Height (in inches)]^2 × 703

> Divide your weight in pounds by the square of your height in inches.

> Then multiply the result by 703.
> Example: Weight: 140 pounds, height: 65 inches
> BMI = $[140 \div (65)^2] \times 703 = 23.29$

Below is a table to help you assess your BMI status.

BMI	Weight Status
Below 18.5	Underweight
18.5–24.9	Normal weight
25.0–29.9	Overweight
30.0 and Above	Obese

BMI is not a perfect tool. It is not a direct measure of body fatness, though it is strongly correlated. An athlete, for example, may have a high BMI, but little body fat. If you need help understanding the significance of your BMI, talk to a member of your health-care team. See chapter 12 for a more in-depth discussion about weight management.

Physical inactivity. It may be that physical activity is the body's greatest medicine. Regular moderate-to-vigorous physical activity helps prevent heart and blood vessel disease, improves insulin sensitivity, aids with weight management, helps control blood cholesterol and blood pressure levels, lowers the risk for cancer and dementia, and so much more. According to the Centers for Disease Control and Prevention (CDC), only 21% of adults in the United States meet recommended levels of physical activity. They advise adults to engage in at least 150 minutes of moderate-intensity aerobic activity such as fast walking and bicycling each week and to perform muscle-strengthening activities like weight lifting at least twice weekly. The CDC guidelines are consistent with the American Diabetes Association guidelines. Learn more about that in chapter 14.

Smoking. If you smoke, try to quit now. Even if you have tried and failed many times, keep trying. If you don't smoke, don't start. People who smoke one pack of cigarettes a day have more than double the heart-attack risk of people who have never smoked. Combined with other risk factors, smoking is even more deadly. Smoking increases the risk of heart disease in many ways:

> Increases blood pressure

> Decreases exercise tolerance

> Increases the tendency for blood to form dangerous clots

> Decreases HDL cholesterol

Chapter 16 covers smoking and smoking cessation in greater detail.

Sleep apnea. According to the American Heart Association, about 20% of adults have at least mild sleep apnea, a condition characterized by heavy snoring and brief periods of not breathing during sleep. This may occur 5–30 or even more times per hour and is strongly linked to high blood pressure, type 2 diabetes, and cardiovascular disease. Sleep apnea and obesity are connected, because excess weight on the upper chest and neck contributes to blocking airflow. If you think you may have sleep apnea or if you feel unrested after sleep, talk to your health-care provider about screening for sleep apnea.

Even without sleep apnea, poor sleep is problematic. Research shows that people who sleep 5 hours or less each day, including naps, are twice as likely to have cardiovascular disease as those who sleep 7 hours per day. Additionally, poor sleep quality appears to boost the risk of developing high blood pressure. Lack of sleep affects blood glucose, too.

Researchers in the Netherlands found that restricting sleep to 4 hours decreased insulin sensitivity by 20–25% compared to sleeping 8.5 hours. If you have trouble falling asleep or staying asleep, be sure to avoid alcohol, caffeine, and large meals several hours before bed. Try relaxing with music, a book, or a warm bath before turning in for the night. Schedule a bedtime and try to stick to it.

Stress. It's unclear how, and even *if*, stress increases the risk of heart disease. It's possible that the body reacts by releasing adrenaline, the "fight or flight" hormone that prepares you to take action against your stressor or danger. In the process, your heart rate and blood pressure may increase. If this continues chronically, it might damage the blood vessel walls. Perhaps more importantly, if reacting to stress takes you away from healthy eating or physical activity, or if it leads you to smoke, it will increase your risk for heart disease and many other problems.

Managing stress can certainly be difficult. Many people find relief in common stress-management techniques such as deep breathing, short exercise breaks, positive self-talk, and meditation. Additionally, living a more relaxed life may be easier if you learn to say "no" more often, get adequate sleep, exercise regularly, eat healthfully, become organized, and make time for the activities and people you enjoy—all things that positively affect you in many ways. Managing stress is also discussed in chapter 19.

Emerging risk factors. Scientists are studying a variety of other possible risk factors or biomarkers, compounds in the body that hint at disease states or risk. One such biomarker that you may have heard of is C-Reactive Protein (CRP). CRP is an indicator of inflammation within the body and may be increased with coronary heart disease. CRP, however, may be elevated for many reasons unrelated to heart disease. Scientists are also looking at the possibility that other inflammatory diseases such as rheumatoid arthritis increase the risk of heart disease. We can expect to learn more about these and other biomarkers and risk factors for heart disease in the years to come.

Take Action

Talk to your health-care provider about your risk for heart disease and stroke. Complete the American Diabetes Association's My Health Advisor survey to calculate your risk for type 2 diabetes, heart disease, and stroke. Find it at diabetes.org/are-you-at-risk/my-health-advisor/.

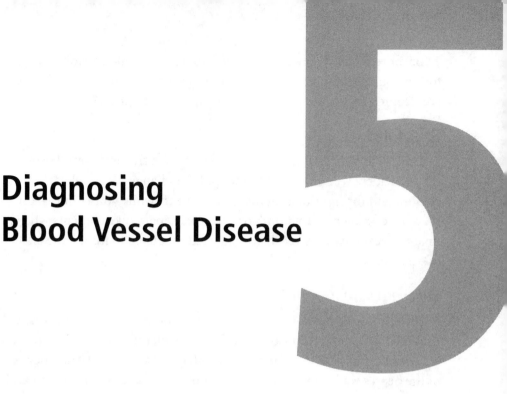

Diagnosing
Blood Vessel Disease

If your health-care provider suspects that you have coronary artery disease or other blood vessel disease, he or she may conduct a variety of tests as well as perform a physical exam and review your medical history, including your blood pressure, blood glucose, and cholesterol levels. You may undergo any of the following tests.

Common Tests to Diagnose Coronary Artery Disease

Electrocardiogram

This test is more commonly called an EKG or an ECG. It records the heart's electrical activity and shows how fast your heart is beating, if it is beating with a regular or irregular rhythm, and the strength and timing of the electrical signals in each part of the heart. Additionally, an ECG can help identify a heart attack in progress or one that has already occurred. This test is typically performed in a health-care provider's office or hospital and takes only a few minutes. A technician will put several electrodes (sticky patches) on your arms, legs, and chest. An ECG is not at all painful.

An ambulatory ECG measures the electrical activity of your heart for

24 or more hours. You will wear a portable device called a Holter monitor, so your health-care provider can see your heart's activity while you are sleeping and while you go about your daily activities.

Stress Test

This is an ECG during exercise, often called a treadmill test. Health-care providers will order this test to look for changes in the electrical rhythm and for signs of ischemia in your heart while you exercise. You may walk or jog on a treadmill or ride a stationary bike. Patients who are unable to exercise may receive an injected medicine to mimic the effects of exercise.

Echocardiogram

An echocardiogram, or "echo," is another noninvasive, painless test. It uses sound waves (ultrasound) to produce pictures of your heart. An echocardiogram can show the size and shape of your heart, the thickness of the heart's walls, how well the heart pumps, problems with valves and blood vessels, and if there are any clots in the chambers of your heart. A technician will put gel on your chest and pass a probe across your chest to produce sound waves that are converted into pictures. An ECG monitors your heart activity. This test takes about an hour and is often done in a clinic or a hospital.

Multidetector Computed Tomography

Multidetector computed tomography (MDCT) is a noninvasive test that uses x-rays to make 3-D images of your heart. It is usually performed in a hospital or clinic. MDCT can show blockages in your coronary arteries, how well your heart pumps blood, the structure of your heart, and abnormalities in your blood vessels. For the test, you will lie down on a table that is connected to the MDCT scanner. A technician will attach electrodes to your chest, because an ECG is also used. The table will move into the machine. The scanner moves around you to get pictures, but it does not touch you. The test is over in about 10 minutes. Sometimes the health-care provider orders this test to be performed with a contrast dye. In this case, the dye is injected through an intravenous (IV) line during the scan.

Radionuclide Angiography

This test is often called a MUGA scan or multi-gated acquisition scan. It is a type of nuclear imaging test and is used to help measure the amount of blood pumped out of the heart during each contraction, identify damage from a previous heart attack, and learn the extent of blockages to the coronary arteries. It can be done at rest or during exercise and is usually performed in a hospital or clinic. During this test, a small amount of a radionuclide or a radioactive substance called a radiopharmaceutical is injected through an IV line. A gamma camera takes images of your heart. This test also makes use of an ECG, so you will have electrodes on your chest, arms, and legs. You will lie down on a table for the resting test. If you are having an exercise test, you will walk on a treadmill or ride a stationary bike and exercise until you've reached your maximum intensity. You'll then move back to the table for the gamma camera to take additional pictures. A MUGA scan is usually over within 2 hours.

Cardiac Catheterization

A cardiac catheterization involves placing a thin, flexible tube, called a catheter, into a blood vessel that leads to the heart. A cardiologist (heart doctor) performs this test in a hospital to check the pressure in the four chambers of your heart, measure the oxygen content of your blood, identify the size and location of plaque in your coronary arteries, and evaluate the function of your heart muscle. You will be awake, but relaxed with the aid of medication. During a cardiac catheterization, the doctor gently guides a catheter from a major blood vessel in your groin, neck, or arm to the heart. A contrast dye can be injected through the catheter. X-rays will then show the dye as it moves through the coronary arteries and identifies areas of blockage. This additional procedure is called a coronary angiography. Depending on what the doctor finds, you may have additional procedures during a cardiac catheterization. Angioplasty is performed when the catheter is used to clear a narrowed or blocked artery. Sometimes the doctor places a wire mesh tube, called a stent, into the blocked area to help keep the blocked area open. The cardiac catheterization can be performed in less than an hour, but you will stay in the hospital for a few hours after the procedure while the hospital staff monitors the bleeding and your pulse and blood pressure.

A Common Test to Diagnose Peripheral Artery Disease

Ankle Brachial Index

Also called ABI, the ankle brachial index is used to diagnose peripheral arterial disease (see chapter 1). While you are lying on your back, a technician measures the blood pressure in your arms and in your ankles, using both a blood pressure cuff and a hand-held ultrasound device. This is a quick procedure and can be performed during a routine medical exam.

Common Tests to Diagnose a Stroke and Blood Vessel Disease in the Brain

Recall from chapter 1 that atherosclerosis in the carotid arteries, called carotid artery disease, can block blood flow to the brain and cause a stroke. This type of stroke is called an ischemic stroke, and it is the most common type. A hemorrhagic stroke occurs when a weakened blood vessel bursts. Below are some common tests to diagnose a stroke.

Brain Computed Tomography

A brain computed tomography (Brain CT) is used to identify bleeding in the brain or damage to the brain cells. A brain CT takes only a few minutes and is performed in a clinic or hospital.

Magnetic Resonance Imaging

Commonly called MRI, this test uses a magnetic field to produce an image of the brain. You will lie on a narrow table that slides into the scanner, which is shaped like a tunnel. Because the MRI uses strong magnets, you may not wear clothing with metal zippers, jewelry, watches, or anything else that contains metal. This test is not painful, though some people are uncomfortable from the loud sounds and from being in a tight space. If you are concerned about being in a small space, ask your health-care provider about open MRI machines or medication to help ease the discomfort of claustrophobia. The test is performed in a clinic or hospital and takes about an hour.

Carotid Angiography

This test is similar to a cardiac catheterization. In carotid angiography, however, the physician places the catheter into the arteries of the brain instead of the arteries of the heart. A contrast dye is injected through the catheter. X-rays will then show the dye as it moves through the arteries and identifies the size and location of blockages. This test is performed in a hospital and takes about an hour. You will need to rest for a few hours after.

Take Action

If your health-care provider recommends any of these tests, ask questions until you understand the purpose of the test, how you will prepare for it, what to expect during and after the test, and when you will receive the results of the test. After you receive the results, ask what this means for you: Are more tests recommended? Will you require medications or a procedure? Do you need a follow-up exam?

A Is for A1C

Do you know your ABCs of diabetes care? You've already learned that diabetes involves more than just blood glucose. Since having diabetes puts you at risk for heart disease, stroke, nerve damage, kidney disease, and more, the American Diabetes Association recommends that you work with your health-care team to manage your ABCs.

A: A1C

B: Blood Pressure

C: Cholesterol

It's important to recognize that each of these is equally important. Often people with diabetes put energy into one at the expense of the others. Sadly, only 19% of Americans with diabetes have each of the three at target levels. Your good health requires you to manage all three. In this chapter, we discuss blood glucose and A1C. Chapters 7 through 10 cover blood pressure and cholesterol.

A1C

When you measure your blood glucose at home or when you go to your health-care provider's office to have it measured, the result shows the concentration of glucose in your blood at just that moment. Not what it was yesterday, what it was an hour ago, or what it might be an hour from now. Blood glucose can be quite volatile, jumping up and down throughout the day. Depending on your habits and how well your diabetes is managed, it can rise a little or a lot. The A1C test gives you and your health-care team a better picture of what's happening with your blood glucose all of those moments you are not measuring it. This simple blood test indicates your average blood glucose level for the past 2–3 months. It's an important test because research has found it is linked to your risk of developing diabetic complications such diseases of the heart, eyes, nerves, and kidneys. The higher the A1C, the greater the risk of complications.

A1C measures the proportion of hemoglobin molecules (the oxygen-carrying protein in your red blood cells) that have glucose attached to them. It's normal to have some sugar-coated hemoglobin, but if you have a lot, it means that your blood glucose has been running high. A1C is expressed as a percent. In someone without diabetes, an A1C might be about 5%. Someone with uncontrolled diabetes might have an A1C of 11%. A typical A1C goal for people with diabetes is 7% or below; however, it varies from person to person.

To help you understand your results, use the table below to convert your A1C to an estimated average glucose (eAG), or go to diabetes.org (diabetes.org/living-with-diabetes/treatment-and-care/blood-glucose-control/a1c/) to use the online Estimated Average Glucose calculator.

Convert Your A1C to an Estimated Average Glucose

A1C (%)	eAG (mg/dl)	A1C (%)	eAG (mg/dl)
5	97	9	212
5.5	111	9.5	226
6	126	10	240
6.5	140	10.5	255
7	154	11	269
7.5	169	11.5	283
8	183	12	298
8.5	197	12.5	312

Target Blood Glucose Goals for Diabetes Management

There is no single number that is ideal for everyone with diabetes. Your health-care provider will help you pick goals based on your age, how long you've had diabetes, your overall health, and other considerations. The following are simply general guidelines for adults. Note that these numbers are not the same values used to diagnose diabetes or prediabetes that are listed in chapter 2.

A1C: <7%

Fasting and Before Meals: 70–130 mg/dl

1–2 Hours After Eating: <180 mg/dl

Monitoring Blood Glucose Is Empowering

Many people with diabetes don't measure their blood glucose because they feel guilty if the number is high or because they don't know what the numbers mean. Some people measure their blood glucose as they were instructed, but make no changes because they don't know how to act on the results. The information you get from self-monitoring blood glucose (SMBG) puts you in control. It tells you if you are making wise food choices, if you need a snack before or after exercise, if you are using the proper amount of insulin, if you're spacing your meals properly, and so much more. The numbers, however, are meaningless and all the strips and lancets you used to measure your blood glucose are wasted if you do nothing with those numbers. Monitoring and interpreting the numbers is the only way to know how your body responds to food, medication, physical activity, illness, and stress. Without SMBG, you are guessing. And you can't make improvements in your diabetes management plan based on a guess.

If you have unexplained high or low readings, try to figure out what caused them. If you don't SMBG or if you do nothing with the results, you have lost an important opportunity to control your diabetes and your health.

Many Things Affect Blood Glucose

Sometimes it's obvious why a blood glucose reading is very high or very low—but not always. If you're unsure, put on your detective hat and consider each of the following.

Food and drink. Carbohydrate has the greatest impact on your blood glucose. Your body digests the carbohydrate-containing foods so that glucose can enter your bloodstream. If you eat a little carbohydrate, your blood sugar will probably go up just a little. But if you eat a lot of carbohydrate, your blood sugar will likely go up a lot. Some foods raise blood

Yikes! My A1C Has Got to Be Wrong!

Lisa measures her blood glucose every morning and just before bed a few times each week. Her fasting blood glucose (first thing in the morning before eating or drinking) is always close to her target and ranges between 95 and 128 mg/dl. Before bed, her blood glucose ranges between 110 and 130 mg/dl. So how could her A1C be 8.5%, an estimated average glucose of 197 mg/dl? She can't even remember a time when her blood glucose meter flashed a number higher than 165. What could be wrong?

Each week, Lisa takes about 10 measurements and feels good about her results, so she never takes additional readings. The A1C, however, reflects the average blood glucose every day, all day. It covers much more than just her 10 data points each week. After receiving her A1C results, Lisa started checking her blood glucose after meals. To her surprise, she saw numbers well over 200 and frequently over 250 mg/dl. Indeed, an A1C of 8.5% accurately described her blood glucose patterns. Lisa worked with a registered dietitian nutritionist (RD or RDN) to create a meal plan that kept her blood glucose levels in a healthy range after eating. The next time her A1C was measured, it was below 7%.

Bob's experience was different. He had such a difficult time controlling his blood glucose. Sometimes it was well over 400 mg/dl, and other times it dropped to 40 mg/dl. Imagine his surprise when his A1C came back at his goal of 7%, an estimated average glucose of 154 mg/dl. How could his A1C be at target range when his blood glucose jumped all over the place throughout the day?

In this case, his large number of hypoglycemic events (low blood glucose) brought his average way down. Bob worked with his physician and registered dietitian nutritionist, who is also a certified diabetes educator, to stabilize his blood glucose. Over the next weeks, he had fewer highs and many fewer lows. He felt healthy for the first time in more than a year.

glucose faster than others. For example, a lot of people find that drinking orange juice raises their blood glucose faster and higher than eating an orange does. This might occur because it takes more time to digest the orange than it does to digest the orange juice. Eating fat or protein at your meal or snack might slow down digestion also and cause blood glucose to rise more slowly. Drinking alcoholic beverages may cause low blood glucose, especially if you drink on an empty stomach.

Insulin and other medications. If you take diabetes medications, how much you take and when you take them affect how your body uses glucose. Taking too much insulin, for example, will likely cause hypoglycemia (low blood glucose). If you take too little, your blood sugar will spike (hyperglycemia). If you take your insulin at the wrong time, your blood glucose may go too low and then too high, or vice versa. Other medications can have similar effects, especially if they are the type of medication that triggers your pancreas to produce more insulin.

Exercise. Being physically active is one of the best ways to be good to yourself. It's important, though, to learn how exercise affects your blood glucose. Typically, it increases insulin sensitivity and helps your muscles pull glucose out of the blood. This is really a good thing, but if you are on insulin or some types of oral medication, you must take caution to avoid hypoglycemia during and after exercise. Sometimes, strenuous exercise temporarily raises blood glucose.

Stress and illness. Emotional stress may or may not cause spikes in blood glucose. Physical stress such as having the flu, lacking sleep, or recovering from surgery frequently elevates blood glucose.

When to Self-Monitor Blood Glucose

In the example with Lisa on page 30, you see that by measuring her blood glucose only before meals and at bedtime, she missed a big part of what was happening. Unfortunately, she didn't even know that there was a problem until she got the results of her A1C test. Below is a sample schedule that can help you identify your blood glucose patterns. Talk to your health-care team to pick the schedule that's right for you. Whatever SMBG schedule you keep, be sure to keep a record, so both you and a member of your health-care team can review it carefully. You may be tempted to simply store the results in your blood glucose meter, but this is rarely enough. It's much more telling and easier to identify patterns if you view the results of several days on paper or on the computer.

	Fasting	2 Hours After Breakfast	Before Lunch	2 Hours After Lunch	Before Dinner	2 Hours After Dinner	Bedtime
Sunday	✓	✓					
Monday			✓	✓			
Tuesday					✓	✓	✓
Wednesday	✓	✓					
Thursday			✓	✓			
Friday					✓	✓	✓
Saturday	✓	✓					

You may wonder why this schedule suggests checking blood glucose both before and after meals. Having both numbers allows you to interpret the data. For example, if your postdinner reading was 215 mg/dl, you might think that it was high because of the food you ate. It's possible, however, that the food had only a small effect and that your blood glucose was already high before you sat down to the table. An after-dinner blood glucose measurement of 215 mg/dl means something very different if your premeal blood glucose is 130 mg/dl than it does if you start your meal at 200 mg/dl.

There are other opportunities to get meaningful numbers. You should also check your blood glucose once in a while at 2 a.m. or 3 a.m., especially if you take insulin, suspect that you experience hypoglycemia while sleeping, or have unexplained hyperglycemia first thing in the morning. Do additional blood glucose checks:

➤ when you feel sick

➤ if you have symptoms of hypoglycemia or if you have trouble recognizing the signs of hypoglycemia

➤ before, during, and after exercise

➤ if you consumed more alcohol than usual

- when you change diabetes medications, dosages of your diabetes medication, or any other medication that can affect blood glucose

- when you change your diet or exercise routine

- if you have gained or lost weight

What Is Hypoglycemia?

Hypoglycemia or low blood glucose is defined as blood glucose below 70 mg/dl. People may experience hypoglycemia with a range of symptoms including shakiness, dizziness, sweating, confusion, anxiousness, rapid heartbeat, irritability, lack of coordination, or even unconsciousness; some may have no symptoms at all. Some people will experience symptoms of hypoglycemia even when their blood glucose is above 70 mg/dl. This is not a reason to worry. It may happen when you are just beginning to get control of your blood glucose, because your body has become accustomed to having a blood glucose of a certain level. Once you've been in control for a longer period of time, you should no longer have symptoms of low blood sugar when you do not have hypoglycemia.

Typically hypoglycemia results from one or more of the following:

- Skipping or delaying a meal or eating too little carbohydrate

- Being more physically active than usual

- Taking too much glucose-lowering medication such as insulin

- Drinking alcohol, especially on an empty stomach or without adequate carbohydrate

The best way to prevent hypoglycemia is to frequently monitor your blood glucose; you will learn how your blood glucose responds to various foods, amounts of food, exercise, and more. Should you experience blood glucose below 70, however, follow the "Rule of 15" to bring it back up.

Step 1: Consume about 15 grams of carbohydrate. Pure glucose in the form of glucose tablets or gel is ideal because it works quickly and contains minimal calories. Other good choices include 1 tablespoon of honey or sugar, 1/2 cup of fruit juice or regular soda,

1 cup of fat-free milk, one small piece of fruit, or 2 tablespoons of raisins. Resist the temptation to consume excess food or carbohydrate, because it usually leads to high blood glucose. And because fat may delay absorption, resist grabbing a candy bar and go for options that only or primarily contain carbohydrate.

Step 2: Sit quietly for 15 minutes. Then check your blood glucose again. If it's still low, consume another 15 grams of carbohydrate.

Step 3: Wait another 15 minutes and check again. Keep doing this until your blood glucose is back in the healthy range.

Step 4: Have a snack if you won't be eating your next meal for an hour or more.

Severe hypoglycemia, especially if you lose consciousness, prevents you from treating yourself, so you may require someone to give you an injection of the hormone glucagon. Warn family and friends that you should not take anything by mouth unless you are conscious and can swallow. If you are at risk for severe hypoglycemia, discuss this with your health-care provider and get a prescription for glucagon. Make sure your friends and family know how to give you this lifesaving injection.

Did You Know?

Hypoglycemia can cause your heart to beat rapidly. If you have heart disease, talk to your health-care provider to learn how low blood glucose might affect you and what precautions you should take.

Be Your Own Detective

Let's say that for fasting and before meals, your blood glucose target is 70–130 mg/dl and that it's <180 mg/dl for 1–2 hours after meals. The following table shows your record for 1 week.

All of these numbers are within your target range except for your postlunch measurements. Each time you measured your blood glucose after lunch, it was higher than your goal. Now you need to figure out why. Did you take your medications improperly or eat too much carbohydrate at lunch? Have you been less active than usual? The solution

	Fasting	2 Hours After Breakfast	Before Lunch	2 Hours After Lunch	Before Dinner	2 Hours After Dinner	Bedtime
Sunday	118	155					
Monday			107	(183)			
Tuesday					130	166	131
Wednesday	101	123	91	(203)			
Thursday					128	155	118
Friday	121	151					
Saturday			101	(206)			

may be to eat a little less carbohydrate at lunch or to take a walk before or after eating. If you can't figure this out on your own, make an appointment with your health-care provider or certified diabetes educator.

Meter Troubleshooting

Sometimes the numbers from a meter don't make much sense because of problems with the meter, the strips, or the user's technique.

> Strips will give an inaccurate reading if they have expired or have been exposed to extreme temperatures or excess humidity. Keep your strips in their original packaging, and don't leave them in your car or in your bathroom.

> Some meters require coding each time you start using a new vial of strips. With some meters, you'll enter a numeric code that you'll find on the packaging for the strips. Other meters require that you insert a chip that comes with each package of strips.

> Having food or dirt on your hands may affect the readings. If you have a shockingly high number, wash your hands and try again. Food residue from your last meal or snack may be the real culprit.

> If you put too little blood on your strip, the result may be a number lower than your actual blood glucose. To obtain a large enough drop of blood, start with warm hands and hold them down at your sides for a few minutes or shake your hands vigorously. Once you have pricked your fingertip, gently massage your finger from knuckle to tip to push the blood out.

Continuous Glucose Monitoring

If you wanted to track your glucose levels every hour for a day, you would need 24 blood glucose strips and 24 drops of blood, and you would need to wake up every hour during the night. Or you could use a continuous glucose monitor (CGM). A CGM allows the user to track glucose levels on a minute-to-minute basis. This information shows important trends such as glucose rising or falling and the response to exercise. It can detect low blood glucose in the middle of the night that would otherwise go undetected. And it can show a better picture of the action of your insulin or other medications. If your glucose is in an unsafe range or if it is dropping rapidly, an alarm can alert you to take action.

A CGM uses a tiny sensor that is inserted under the skin for several days before needing to be replaced. This sensor checks glucose levels in the fluid around your cells rather than in your blood. A transmitter sends information about your glucose levels to a wireless monitor. Using a CGM doesn't allow you to get rid of your blood glucose meter, though. You will still need blood glucose measurements to calibrate the CGM and to verify glucose levels before taking corrective action. A big drawback to the CGM is its expense. Typically, insurance companies authorize continuous glucose monitors only for people who take insulin. However, some medical practices may be able to send you home with one for a couple of days.

Take Action

If you don't already know, ask your health-care provider what your target blood glucose levels are for various times of the day. Discuss the appropriate schedule to self-monitoring your blood glucose. Don't simply record the results. Ask for help if you don't understand them. Then, with the help of a member of your health-care team, make the appropriate changes to your diabetes treatment plan.

B Is for Blood Pressure

One in every three American adults has high blood pressure or hypertension, but it affects the majority of people with diabetes. Do you know if you have high blood pressure? According to the Centers for Disease Control and Prevention, about 20% of American adults with high blood pressure don't even know they have it. Equally disturbing is that only 47% of people with high blood pressure have it under control well enough to minimize the health risk.

Hypertension can have devastating effects on many organs and body systems, including the blood vessels, heart, kidneys, and eyes. It contributes to nearly 1,000 deaths per day. Many people aren't aware that they have hypertension, or that it's poorly controlled, because there are usually no symptoms. For this reason, and because it is so deadly, hypertension is dubbed the "silent killer."

Many factors contribute to high blood pressure. As we age, our blood vessels lose flexibility. High blood pressure is more common in men and in African-Americans. Not only is high blood pressure more likely to affect African-Americans, it usually develops at an earlier age in that group and is more severe. These are not things that you have control over, but you do have some control over other contributing factors, including inactivity, poor diet, overweight and obesity, insulin resistance, tobacco use, and excessive alcohol intake.

What Is Blood Pressure?

Blood pressure is the pressure or force of blood against the artery walls. It is recorded as two numbers and is given in units of mm Hg (millimeters of mercury).

> *Systolic blood pressure* is the first or top number. It is the pressure of the blood on the artery walls as the blood is pushed out of the heart.

> *Diastolic blood pressure* is the second or bottom number. It is the pressure on the artery walls between heartbeats, when the heart muscle is resting and refilling with blood. Diastolic blood pressure is lower than the systolic blood pressure.

Just as your blood glucose varies over the day, blood pressure goes up and down as well. This is normal as long as it stays within a healthy range. Sleep, stress, your posture, physical activity, and more factors affect your blood pressure.

High Blood Pressure Ravages the Body

Healthy arteries relax and stretch as necessary to allow blood to pass through unhindered. If the pressure on the artery walls is chronically high, the arteries become overstretched. Damage occurs to more than just the heart. Often the risk of these health problems is greater when high blood pressure is combined with diabetes. Here's what can happen:

> *Blood vessel damage and atherosclerosis.* The excess pressure damages the endothelium, making it more permeable to LDL cholesterol and other harmful substances.

> *Aneurysm.* The constant pressure can cause a section of a weakened artery to bulge. If the bulge or aneurysm ruptures, it can cause life-threatening bleeding or death. If an aneurysm occurs in the brain, it can cause a stroke.

> *Enlarged left heart (left ventricular hypertrophy).* The heart is forced to work harder because of the increased pressure or resistance, which causes the left ventricle of the heart to enlarge and stiffen.

This increases your risk of heart attack, heart failure, and sudden cardiac death.

➤ *Heart failure.* Persistent strain on the heart weakens the heart muscle.

➤ *Stroke.* Brain cells can die when chronic high blood pressure weakens a blood vessel to the brain and causes the blood vessel to narrow or rupture. Strokes also occur when plaque in the brain's arteries breaks off and forms a clot.

➤ *Vascular dementia.* Blocked blood flow to the brain can cause problems with memory, reasoning, judgment, and more. The impairment can range from mild to severe. People with diabetes are at increased risk of vascular dementia.

➤ *Kidney damage.* Your kidneys need healthy blood vessels to filter blood, but excess pressure can damage the blood vessels leading to and within the kidneys. High blood pressure can also cause an aneurysm in a blood vessel leading to the kidney.

➤ *Eye damage.* Damage to the vessels that supply blood to the retina can cause bleeding in the eye, blurred vision, and blindness.

➤ *Sexual dysfunction.* If damage occurs to the blood vessels that supply the sexual organs, men may experience erectile dysfunction (the inability to have or maintain an erection), and women may experience low sexual desire.

Classification of Blood Pressure for Adults

Blood Pressure Classification	Systolic Blood Pressure: top number (mmHg)	Diastolic Blood Pressure: bottom number (mmHg)
Normal	<120	*and* <80
Prehypertension	120–139	*or* 80–89
Hypertension Stage 1	140–159	*or* 90–99
Hypertension Stage 2	>160	*or* >100

Source: *The Seventh Report of the Joint National Committee on Prevention, Detection, Evaluation, and Treatment of High Blood Pressure*

Know Your Numbers

Have your blood pressure checked at every routine medical visit. A trained person should measure your blood pressure after you've sat quietly for 5 minutes. Your arm should be supported at the level of your heart.

Classification of hypertension is based on the systolic *or* the diastolic number. It is not necessary for both numbers to be elevated to have the diagnosis of prehypertension or hypertension. For example, if your blood pressure is 115/88 mmHg, you have prehypertension, because the diastolic number is between 80 and 89 mmHg even though your systolic number is in the normal range. Likewise, if your blood pressure is 144/82 mmHg, you have hypertension stage 1, because your systolic number falls in that category even though your diastolic number falls in a lower category.

Prehypertension is reason to take action. The higher your blood pressure, the greater is your risk of heart attack, heart failure, stroke, and kidney disease. Do not wait until you have been diagnosed with high blood pressure before talking to your health-care team about both your risk and the actions you should take to protect your health. If you are between 40 and 70 years of age, beginning with blood pressure of 115/75 mmHg, each increment of 20 mmHg in systolic blood pressure or 10 mmHg in diastolic blood pressure doubles your risk of cardiovascular disease.

You cannot be diagnosed with high blood pressure from a single measurement. If your blood pressure is elevated, your health-care provider will ask you to return to the office to have it measured again. You might also be instructed to monitor your blood pressure at home with an electronic blood pressure machine or to use an ambulatory blood pressure monitor that automatically takes your blood pressure several times over a 24-hour period. This allows your health-care provider to assess your blood pressure over an entire day.

American Diabetes Association's Blood Pressure Goals

The ADA recommends that people with both diabetes and hypertension achieve blood pressure <140/80 mmHg through a combination of lifestyle changes and medications as needed.

Lifestyle Changes to Improve Blood Pressure Levels

Lowering elevated blood pressure and keeping it lowered is hugely beneficial. In a large study of people with type 2 diabetes, lowering blood pressure to an average of 144/82 mmHg significantly reduced the incidence of stroke, diabetes-related death, heart failure, vision loss, and microvascular complications such as kidney disease.

In addition to taking medications as prescribed, you can do a lot of things to improve your blood pressure, and reduce your risk for heart disease and all of the other health problems noted above. If the following list seems overwhelming, pick just one thing to work on, then another, then another, and so on. You will learn more about these lifestyle changes in later chapters.

➤ Stop smoking.

➤ Be physically active most days of the week.

➤ If you are overweight, lose at least a few pounds.

➤ Reduce your sodium intake.

➤ Drink alcohol in moderation, if at all.

➤ Eat plenty of fruits, vegetables, beans and fiber-rich grains.

➤ Manage stress.

White-Coat Hypertension

Margie was surprised when the nurse told her that her blood pressure was high, so she asked the nurse to measure it again. Periodically Margie measures her own blood pressure when she visits her dad, who has a home blood pressure monitor. Margie's blood pressure had never been elevated at her dad's place, so she was certain that it was a mistake this time. When the nurse measured it again a few minutes later, Margie's blood pressure remained elevated. Her doctor sent her home with instructions to use a home blood pressure monitor twice a day for the next 2 weeks. Margie returned with a record of her blood pressure measurements, and all were in a healthy range. Again to Margie's surprise, her blood pressure was elevated in the doctor's office. The doctor suspects that Margie has white-coat hypertension, so called because blood pressure is elevated only at the doctor's office (and because health-care professionals frequently wear white coats). Both Margie and her doctor will continue to monitor her blood pressure. Research suggests that individuals with white-coat hypertension are at high risk for developing sustained hypertension.

Medications

Diet and lifestyle changes are your first line of defense. However, they don't always do enough. Medications work in conjunction with diet, exercise, and other heart-healthy behaviors. Frequently, people with hypertension need more than one medication to sufficiently reduce their blood pressure. Talk to your health-care provider and pharmacist about your medications. You should know the purpose of the medication, when to take it, the proper dosage, if it is better taken with food or without, what to do if you miss a dose, the side effects you should watch for, and if you should be aware of any potential interactions with food, supplements, or other medications.

Blood Pressure–Lowering Medications

Type of Drug	Common Names	Actions
Diuretics	Bumetanide (Bumex)	Helps the kidneys remove excess fluid from your body and excrete it through the urine.
	Chlorthalidone (Hygroton)	
	Chlorothiazide (Diuril)	
	Furosemide (Lasix)	
	Metolazone (Mykrox, Zaroxolyn)	
	Hydrochlorothiazide (Esidrix, Hydrodiuril, Microzide)	
	Spironolactone (Aldactone)	
Beta-blockers	Acebutolol (Sectral)	Reduces heart rate and the heart's workload.
	Atenolol (Tenormin)	May mask the symptoms of hypoglycemia.
	Bisoprolol fumarate (Zebeta)	
	Metoprolol tartrate (Lopressor)	
	Metoprolol succinate (Toprol-XL)	
	Nadolol (Corgard)	
	Propranolol hydrochloride (Inderal)	

*Not a complete list

Type of Drug	Common Names	Actions
ACE-inhibitors	Benazepril hydrochloride (Lotensin) Captopril (Capoten) Enalapril maleate (Vasotec) Fosinopril sodium (Monopril) Lisinopril (Prinivel, Zestril) Quinapril hydrochloride (Accupril) Ramipril (Altace)	Helps relax the blood vessels by inhibiting the production of a substance that narrows the blood vessels. Reduces the risk of diabetes-related kidney disease.
Angiotensin II receptor block-ers (ARBs)	Candesartan (Atacand) Eprosartan mesylate (Teveten) Irbesarten (Avapro) Losartan potassium (Cozaar) Telmisartan (Micardis) Valsartan (Diovan)	Helps the blood vessels to relax by blocking the production of a compound necessary to constrict the blood vessels. Reduces the risk of diabetes-related kidney disease.
Calcium-chan-nel blockers	Amlodipine besylate (Norvasc, Lotrel) Diltiazem hydrochloride (Cardizem, Tiazac) Felodipine (Plendil) Isradipine (DynaCirc) Nicardipine (Cardene) Nifedipine (Adalat, Procardia) Nisoldipine (Sular) Verapamil hydrochloride (Calan, Covera HS, Verelan)	Reduces the force of the heart's contraction by block-ing calcium from entering the smooth muscle cells of the heart and arteries.
Alpha-blockers	Doxazosin mesylate (Cardura) Prazosin hydrochloride (Minipress) Terazosin hydrochloride (Hytrin)	Relaxes the muscle tone of the blood vessel walls.

*Not a complete list

Take Action

If prescribed, take your blood pressure medications appropriately. Ask to have your blood pressure measured at every appointment with your health-care provider, and talk to your health-care provider about the steps you can take to improve your blood pressure or to lower your risk of developing high blood pressure.

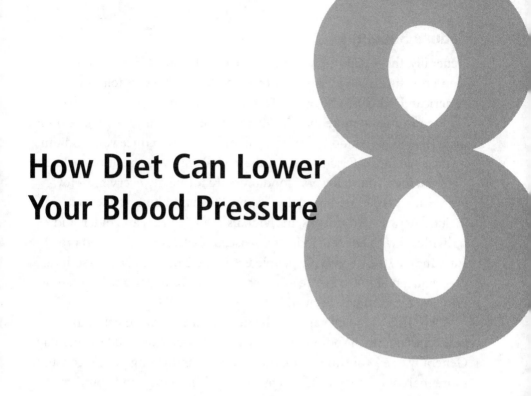

How Diet Can Lower Your Blood Pressure

You have a lot of control over your blood pressure. According to the National Heart, Lung, and Blood Institute, each of the following actions is significantly helpful. And of course, take your medications as prescribed.

Diet and Lifestyle Modification	Approximate Lowering of Systolic Blood Pressure
Lose weight.	5–20 mmHg for 22-pound weight loss
Engage in regular cardiovascular activity, such as brisk walking, for at least 30 minutes on most days of the week.	4–9 mmHg
Limit alcohol to one drink per day for women and two drinks per day for men.	2–4 mmHg
Reduce sodium to ≤2400 mg/day.	2–8 mmHg
Consume a DASH eating plan, a diet rich in fruits, vegetables, and low-fat dairy products and low in saturated fat (see below for a discussion about DASH).	8–14 mmHg

This chapter discusses sodium reduction and the Dietary Approaches to Stop Hypertension (DASH) eating plan.

Reduce Sodium

Generally, the higher the sodium in the diet, the greater is the individual's blood pressure. And as sodium decreases, blood pressure follows. The American Diabetes Association recommends that individuals with diabetes consume no more than 2,300 mg of sodium daily. If you have both diabetes and high blood pressure, you may need to reduce your sodium intake even more. Discuss your sodium goal with your health-care team.

Reducing sodium lowers blood pressure for nearly everyone. However, some people are especially responsive to a sodium reduction. They include African-Americans, individuals aged 51 years and older, and individuals with chronic kidney disease, diabetes, or high blood pressure. In one study involving people with type 2 diabetes, a low-sodium diet reduced blood pressure as much as if a second blood pressure–lowering medication had been added.

According to the Dietary Guidelines for Americans, most of us consume too much sodium, with an average intake of 3,400 mg per day. Generally, men consume more than women, and young people consume more than older people. This is probably because men and younger people typically consume more food than women and older people.

Trimming sodium from your diet requires a lot more than hiding the saltshaker. That's because only about 11% of our sodium intake comes from salt that is added while cooking or at the table. Packaged foods and restaurant foods give us a whopping 77% of our sodium. The remaining 12% comes from sodium that occurs naturally in foods.

As you would expect, high-sodium foods contribute to our excess sodium intake, but so do foods of only moderate sodium content because we eat them so frequently. In fact, the number one contributor of sodium to the diets of Americans is bread. We have toast for breakfast, sandwiches for lunch, and dinner rolls for dinner. If you consume bread often, it's wise to look for lower-sodium options. For that matter, you should look for lower-sodium options of any food you eat frequently. After bread, the top contributors of sodium are chicken and chicken dishes, pizza, and pasta dishes.

Here are few ways to slash sodium from your diet.

➤ Prepare more foods at home and from scratch. Consume more fruits and vegetables because they are naturally low in sodium and rich in potassium, a mineral important for blood pressure control.

➤ Don't add salt to cooking water.

➤ Review the nutrition facts panel on packaged foods. Compare various brands of breads, soups, pasta sauces, cheese, etc.

➤ Cook with less salt and with more sodium-free herbs and spices. When purchasing spice blends, read the labels to be certain that salt is not one of the ingredients. Add flavor with vinegars and citrus juices and peels.

➤ Buy canned foods labeled "no salt added." If your family isn't ready for these, mix a can of regular and a can of no salt added together to cut the sodium by almost half.

➤ Rinse canned beans, corn, and other vegetables.

➤ Don't forget to consider the sodium content of beverages and condiments.

➤ When eating in restaurants, ask for lower-sodium options. Visit Healthy Dining Finder at healthydiningfinder.com to search for local and chain restaurants that meet specific nutrition guidelines.

Sodium Shockers and Surprises

Food	Sodium Content (mg)
Salt, 1 teaspoon	2,325
Whole wheat bread, 1 slice	146
Bagel, plain, 4 1/2 inch	700
Grilled chicken fillet sandwich	982
Kidney beans, 1/2 cup canned, drained and rinsed	165
Brown rice, 1/2 cup cooked	5
Rice pilaf, packaged, 1/2 cup cooked	512
Seasoned bread crumbs, 1/4 cup	400
American cheese, processed, 1 ounce	468
Light yogurt, strawberry, 8-ounce container	132
Salted peanuts, 1 ounce (about 1/4 cup)	189
Instant chocolate pudding, 1/2 cup	417

Source: USDA Nutrient Data Laboratory

- Retrain your taste buds. You can learn to prefer lower-sodium foods. Just start eating them. If you're having trouble, make the changes gradually.

- Use only half or one-quarter of seasoning packets that come with rice and other packaged foods.

- Don't rely on your sense of taste to tell you if a food is salty. For example, a 1/2 cup serving of instant chocolate pudding contains 417 mg of sodium, more than twice the sodium in a 1-ounce serving of salted peanuts.

- Before using a potassium-based salt substitute, check with your health-care team. This is a great choice for some people, but not for everyone, depending on the individual's health conditions and medications.

Do You Know the Difference Between Sodium and Salt?

Even though the two words are often used as if they mean the same thing, they do not. Sodium is a mineral. The body requires it in small amounts. Table salt is a combination of sodium and chloride, another mineral. One teaspoon of salt contains 2,325 mg of sodium—the limit (or more) for an entire day!

The DASH Diet

Research funded by the National Heart, Lung, and Blood Institute (NHLBI) showed that changing diet can lower blood pressure as well as a single drug might! The DASH (Dietary Approaches to Stop Hypertension) eating pattern is rich in fruits, vegetables, and low-fat or nonfat dairy products. It also includes whole grains, nuts, fish, poultry, oils, and soft fats. It limits red and processed meats, sugary drinks, sweets, and solid fats. Even without losing weight or restricting sodium, study subjects experienced a significant improvement in both their systolic and diastolic blood pressures.

The first DASH study compared three eating plans: a typical American diet, which is high in unhealthful saturated fats and added sugars and low in whole grains and other plant foods; a typical American diet with additional fruits and vegetables; and the DASH eating plan as described above. The results were dramatic. The diet high in fruits and vegetables lowered blood pressure, but the DASH plan lowered it even more. When researchers added a sodium restriction to the DASH diet, the results got even better.

To what does DASH owe its success? DASH is rich in a trifecta of minerals: potassium, calcium, and magnesium. The foods provide ample fiber and little saturated fats, trans fats, and added sugars. This combination is much greater than the individual foods or nutrients.

The DASH Eating Plan

This table describes the DASH eating plan at two different calorie levels. You can see a description of the plan at calorie levels ranging from 1,200 to 3,100 at the NHLBI website (nhlbi.nih.gov/health/health-topics/topics/dash/followdash.html).

Food Group	Daily Servings on 1,600 Calorie Diet	Daily Servings on 2,000 Calorie Diet	Examples
Grains, mostly whole	6	6–8	1 slice whole wheat bread
			1/2 cup cooked rice, pasta, oatmeal
Vegetables	3–4	4–5	1 cup raw lettuce, kale, spinach, or other leafy vegetable
			1/2 cup cut-up raw or cooked vegetable
			1/2 cup tomato or other vegetable juice
Fruit	4	4–5	1 medium fruit such as apple, pear, plum, orange, and peach
			1/4 cup dried fruit such as raisins and prunes
			1/2 cup fresh, frozen, or canned fruit
			1/2 cup 100% fruit juice
Fat-free or low-fat milk products	2–3	2–3	1 cup milk or yogurt
			1 1/2 ounces cheese

Food Group	Daily Servings on 1,600 Calorie Diet	Daily Servings on 2,000 Calorie Diet	Examples
Lean meats, poultry, and fish	4 or less	6 or less	1 ounce cooked lean beef, lamb, pork, poultry, or fish 1 whole egg 2 egg whites
Nuts, seeds, and legumes	3–4 per week	4–5 per week	1/3 cup or 1 1/2 ounces nuts 2 Tbsp or 1/2 ounce seeds 2 Tbsp peanut or almond butter 1/2 cup cooked dried beans and peas (legumes)
Fats and oils	2	2–3	1 tsp soft margarine 1 tsp vegetable oil 1 Tbsp salad dressing 2 Tbsp light salad dressing
Sweets and added sugars	3 or less per week	5 or less per week	1 Tbsp sugar, jelly, maple syrup 1/2 cup sorbet 1 cup lemonade
Sodium	2,300 mg or less per day	2,300 mg or less per day	

DASH Beyond Blood Pressure

DASH can do even more than lower blood pressure. Additional research has found that this eating pattern may also improve bone health, reduce the risk of kidney stones and colorectal cancer, improve HDL cholesterol, lower triglycerides, and improve insulin sensitivity.

DASH and Diabetes

If you're concerned that a DASH eating style may not be a good fit for people with diabetes, you'll be comforted to know that in a small study, people with type 2 diabetes who followed the DASH diet benefited in many ways. They experienced weight loss, smaller waist circumferences, lower fasting glucose and A1C levels, reduced blood pressure, and improved HDL and LDL cholesterol levels. Recent studies have modified the DASH diet to include additional unsaturated fats or protein. The modified diets also lowered blood pressure, improved cholesterol, and reduced cardiovascular risk.

Before changing your diet, it's wise to check with your health-care provider. And when you start your new diet plan, measure your blood glucose more often, especially before and after meals.

Take Action

Identify places in your diet to reduce your sodium intake. Look for recipes that boost flavor with herbs and spices instead of salt. Eat fruits and/or vegetables at every meal and snack. Ask for a referral to a registered dietitian nutritionist to help you implement an eating style that is appropriate for you.

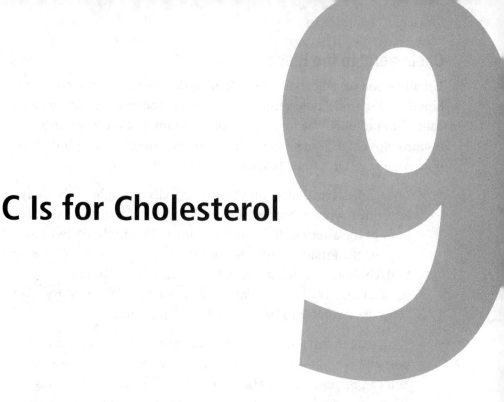

C Is for Cholesterol

Many things may cause or contribute to abnormal cholesterol levels in the blood. These include genetics, poor diet, obesity, poor diabetes control, insulin resistance, medications, and thyroid disorders. Though you can do nothing about your genetics, you can work with your health-care team on each of the other potential contributors to abnormal blood levels.

Functions of Cholesterol

Many people think that cholesterol is all bad. However, if you had no cholesterol in your body, you would be a plant! All animals have cholesterol; no plants do. Cholesterol in the human body is critically important. It is an integral part of every cell membrane, helping to maintain the integrity of the membrane and regulate the passage of compounds in and out of the cell. Cholesterol is necessary for the synthesis of bile acids, which are necessary for fat digestion. The body also uses cholesterol to make vitamin D and some hormones, including estrogen, testosterone, and cortisol.

Cholesterol in the Blood

Usually when we talk about cholesterol in the body, we're referring to blood cholesterol. Cholesterol travels in the blood wrapped in packages called lipoproteins. The main lipoproteins of interest are low-density lipoproteins (LDL), frequently called bad cholesterol, and high-density lipoproteins (HDL), frequently called good cholesterol.

➤ LDL cholesterol delivers cholesterol to cells throughout the body. It is harmful when it burrows below the endothelium into the intimal layer of the artery wall. There it becomes chemically altered and triggers the inflammatory and atherosclerotic processes. Generally, LDL cholesterol is the primary target for therapy. You can remember that LDL is the "bad" kind by associating "L" with "lousy" and "low." It's desirable to have a low LDL measurement.

➤ HDL cholesterol removes cholesterol from the arteries and transports it back to the liver, where it can be recycled or disposed of. You can remember that HDL is the "good" kind by associating "H" with "healthy" and "high." It's desirable to have a high HDL measurement.

Know Your Numbers

The American Diabetes Association recommends that adults with diabetes have a lipid panel (also called a lipoprotein profile) measured each year. *Lipids* is a word used to describe fats. The simple blood test measures triglycerides in the blood as well as cholesterol.

Lipid Panel

Lipid	ADA's Target for Most People with Diabetes
LDL cholesterol	<100 mg/dl
	<70 mg/dl for people with overt CVD
HDL cholesterol	>40 mg/dl in men
	>50 mg/dl in women
Triglycerides	<150 mg/dl

Source: American Diabetes Association Clinical Practice Recommendations (2014)

Before having a lipid panel, you should not eat or drink anything other than water for 9–12 hours. Often health-care providers look at numbers other than LDL cholesterol, HDL cholesterol, and triglycerides. You may see the following on your lab report:

> Total cholesterol: This includes LDL plus HDL cholesterol as well as very low-density lipoprotein (VLDL) cholesterol, a third type of lipoprotein in the blood. According to the American Heart Association, it's desirable to have a total cholesterol level of less than 200 mg/dl.

> Total cholesterol-to-HDL-cholesterol ratio: To determine this ratio, divide your total cholesterol number by your HDL cholesterol number.
>   Total cholesterol ÷ HDL cholesterol
>   Example: Total cholesterol = 200 mg/dl and HDL cholesterol = 50 mg/dl
> $200 ÷ 50 = 4$ (ratio = 4:1)
> A low ratio is best. According to the American Heart Association, an acceptable ratio is below 5:1, but the optimal ratio is 3.5:1.

Size Matters

LDL particles don't come in one size. You may have a lot of big, fluffy, less-damaging LDL particles, or you might have more small, tight, and dense LDL particles that more easily slip into the artery wall and set off the process of building up plaque. Sometimes, to get a greater picture of a patient's risk for cardiovascular disease, a health-care provider will order a blood test that examines the LDL particle size. However, the American Diabetes Association, the American Heart Association, and the American College of Cardiology Foundation have stated that for individuals without symptoms, tests beyond a standard fasting lipid profile are unnecessary to establish an individual's risk for cardiovascular disease.

Where Cholesterol Comes From

We consume cholesterol every time we eat an egg or a cheeseburger or drink a glass of 1% milk. Whenever we eat animal fats, we ingest cholesterol. The current recommendation is that people with (or who are at high risk for developing) cardiovascular disease and type 2 diabetes consume no more than 200 mg of cholesterol per day. For the general population, experts recommend no more than 300 mg of dietary cholesterol per day. Dietary cholesterol, however, is not the major source of cholesterol in our blood. Our bodies make more than enough. Even if we consumed no cholesterol at all, we would have ample cholesterol for our cell membranes, to produce hormones and vitamin D, and for every other function of cholesterol. The amount of saturated and trans fats that you eat affects your blood cholesterol levels more than anything else in your diet. More on that in chapter 10.

Common Sources of Dietary Cholesterol

Food	Cholesterol (mg)
Egg, 1	185
Bacon & egg biscuit, 1	352
Hamburger patty, 85% lean, 4 ounces	102
Salmon, cooked, 4 ounces	71
Whole milk, 1 cup	24
2% milk, 1 cup	20
Cheddar cheese, 1 ounce	30
Corn muffin, 1 medium	29

Source: USDA Nutrient Data Laboratory

Lifestyle Changes to Improve Cholesterol Levels

Many things can improve your lipid levels and lower your risk for heart disease. You saw many of these behaviors on the list of lifestyle changes that can improve blood pressure. In fact, these behaviors will improve your health in multiple ways beyond lowering your risk for heart disease.

➤ Stop smoking.

➤ Be physically active most days of the week.

➤ If you are overweight, lose at least a few pounds.

- Replace saturated fats with monounsaturated and polyunsaturated fats.

- Reduce your cholesterol intake.

- Avoid trans fats.

- Drink alcohol in moderation, if at all.

- Eat plenty of fruits, vegetables, beans, and fiber-rich grains.

Medications

As with elevated blood pressure, diet and lifestyle changes are the cornerstone of your treatment plan to improve your lipids. However, taking medications is frequently necessary. Usually, the treatment of elevated LDL cholesterol is considered to have first priority. Talk to your healthcare provider and pharmacist to learn how your medications work and how you should take them.

Lipid Therapy Medications

Type of Drug	Common Names	Actions
Statins (HMG CoA reductase inhibitors)	Atorvastatin (Lipitor) Fluvastatin (Lescol) Lovastatin (Mevacor, Altoprev) Pravastatin (Pravachol) Rosuvastatin Calcium (Crestor) Simvastatin (Zocor)	Works in the liver to prevent the formation of cholesterol and increases the removal of LDL cholesterol by the liver. Targets LDL cholesterol. Offers moderate improvements on triglycerides and HDL cholesterol.
Selective cholesterol absorption inhibitors	Ezetimibe (Zetia)	Prevents the absorption of cholesterol from the intestine. Targets LDL cholesterol. Offers moderate improvements on triglycerides and HDL cholesterol.

*Not a complete list

Type of Drug	Common Names	Actions
Resins (bile acid sequestrants)	Cholestyramine (Questran, Questran Light, Prevalite, Locholest, Locholest Light) Colestipol (Colestid) Colesevelam HCl (WelChol)	These medicines bind to bile, making it unavailable for digestion. More bile must be made and in the process, additional cholesterol is used up. Targets LDL cholesterol. Colesevelam HCl , sold under the brand name WelChol, is also sometimes used to lower blood glucose in people with type 2 diabetes.
Fibrates	Gemfibrozil (Lopid) Fenofibrate (Antara, Lofibra, Tricor, Triglide) Clofibrate (Atromid-S)	Targets triglycerides. May improve HDL cholesterol levels.
Niacin (nicotinic acid)	Niacin (Niaspan)	Acts on the liver to increase HDL cholesterol and to lower triglycerides and LDL cholesterol. Considered to be the most effective drug for raising HDL cholesterol. May raise blood glucose levels. Use only prescription niacin to treat abnormal lipid levels.

*Not a complete list

Why Does LDL Get So Much Attention?

The answer to this is simple. Most of the research points to LDL cholesterol as the most important lipid target because of its role in atherosclerosis. Fortunately, many heart-healthy lifestyle behaviors improve LDL cholesterol as well as total and HDL cholesterol and triglycerides.

Take Action

Ask for a lipid panel if you have not had one in the last 12 months. Review your results with a member of your health-care team. If prescribed, take your cholesterol-lowering medications appropriately.

Dietary Fats Affect Your Cholesterol Levels

There is no reason to fear dietary fat, but many people do.

Myth: Eating fat makes you fat.
Truth: Fat contains a lot of calories (9 calories per gram), and eating too many calories packs on the pounds. Fats can and should be a part of your healthy diet, however.

Myth: Eating fat clogs arteries.
Truth: Eating too many unhealthy fats (saturated and trans fats) increases blood lipids, which raises your risk for atherosclerosis and heart disease. It's smart to eat a source of the healthy monounsaturated and polyunsaturated fats at each meal (see below for more information).

Roles of Dietary Fats

Fat makes our food taste good, and it gives the food a wonderful, creamy texture and mouth feel. It makes food moist and aids in browning. But dietary fats play important roles beyond making food desirable. Fats in the diet also dissolve and carry fat-soluble nutrients such as some vitamins and disease-fighting compounds like the carotenoids beta-carotene and lycopene. This helps us absorb them.

For example, researchers gave study participants salads with fat-free dressing, reduced-fat dressing, and full-fat dressing. The researchers detected only tiny amounts of absorbed carotenoids in the participants' blood after they ate the salad with fat-free dressing. The study participants absorbed a more noticeable amount of carotenoids when they consumed the reduced-fat dressing and even more with the full-fat salad dressing.

Additionally, dietary fats supply the body with two fatty acids the body needs but cannot make. Finally, many people find that eating a bit of fat at meals helps them to stay full longer.

Types of Dietary Fatty Acids

In general, Americans eat an appropriate amount of fat, yet our choices of fats and fat-containing foods are often not ideal. Research suggests that the *types* of fatty acids consumed more greatly influence cardiovascular risk than does the *amount* of fat in the diet. About 34% of our calories come from fat. Federal guidelines suggest that we eat 20–35% of our calories in the form of fat, so many people are on target for total fat. The unhealthful saturated fatty acids, however, are too prominent in our diets and contribute about 11% of our total calories.

The American Diabetes Association recommends consuming no more than 10% of total calories as saturated fats. Guidelines issued by the American Heart Association in 2013 recommend even stricter limits for individuals with elevated LDL cholesterol levels. These individuals should limit saturated fat to just 5–6% of total calories.

Trans fatty acids are also harmful, and we should eat as little as possible. Experts recommend that we reduce our saturated fat intake by replacing some with the healthful monounsaturated and polyunsaturated fatty acids. Each type of fatty acid is discussed below and briefly summarized in the following table.

Saturated fats. Aim for as little saturated fat as possible while still enjoying a varied diet of healthful foods. To consume no more than 5–10% of your calories as saturated fat, limit saturated fat intake to 11–22 grams daily if you consume a diet of about 2,000 calories. If your diet is only about 1,400 calories, your saturated fat goal should be no more than 8–16 grams daily. It's very easy to splurge on a dessert or a restaurant meal and find that you've consumed enough

Fatty Acid	Role in Health
Saturated	Increases risk of CVD.
	Raises total cholesterol and LDL cholesterol.
	Decreases insulin sensitivity among people with diabetes and healthy individuals.
Trans	Increases risk of CVD.
	Raises total cholesterol and LDL cholesterol.
	May lower HDL cholesterol.
Monounsaturated	Decreases risk of both CVD and type 2 diabetes.
	When replacing saturated fatty acids, they decrease total cholesterol and LDL cholesterol and improve insulin resistance.
Polyunsaturated Omega-6 Omega-3	Decreases risk of CVD.
	When replacing saturated fatty acids, they decrease total cholesterol, LDL cholesterol, triglycerides, insulin resistance and markers of inflammation.

*Not a complete list

saturated fat for 2 days! (See Common Sources of Saturated Fat below.) Even a single meal very high in saturated fat may harm the blood vessels.

Typically, you can identify foods rich in unhealthful fats by their firmness at room temperature. Consider bacon grease. What happens to it when the pan cools? It becomes solid, giving you a hint that bacon and bacon grease are rich in saturated fats. Lard, beef fat, and butter are also firm at room temperature and are high in saturated fatty acids.

Common Sources of Saturated Fat

Food & Serving Size	Saturated Fat (g)
Whole milk, 1 cup	5
American cheese, 1 ounce	5
Bacon, cooked, 2 slices	3
Chicken nuggets, 6 pieces	3
Beef brisket, cooked, 4 ounces	8
Kielbasa, pan-fried, 1 link (13 ounces)	35
Cheesecake, 1 slice (4 ounces)	12

Source: USDA Nutrient Data Laboratory

Dairy fat and the tropical oils (coconut, palm, and palm kernel), however, are also largely saturated even though they are not solid at room temperature.

Trans fats. To increase the shelf life of processed foods such as crackers, snack cakes, and granola bars, food manufacturers frequently put hydrogenated oils in the food. Hydrogenation converts the healthful unsaturated fatty acids into saturated or trans fatty acids.

Experts recommend that we keep our trans fatty acid intake to less than 1% of total calories (about 1 1/2 grams if consuming 1,400 calories or 2 grams if consuming 2,000 calories daily). This may be harder than you realize, because many packaged foods labeled "No Trans Fats" actually contain traces of these artery-damaging fats. That's because a food may contain up to 0.49 grams of trans fat per serving and still claim zero. If you eat a few servings of food each day with traces of trans fats, you can easily exceed your trans fat limit. Identify minute amounts of trans fats by looking for the words *partially hydrogenated oil* in the ingredients list. There will be at least traces of trans fat present. When oils are fully hydrogenated, they will not contain trans fats. Instead, the unsaturated fatty acids have been converted to saturated fatty acids.

Your best strategy to avoid trans fats and excess saturated fats is to limit highly processed foods and consume more fruits, vegetables, and unprocessed or minimally processed grains. The U.S. Food and Drug Administration has proposed a ban on partially hydrogenated oils. Should this take place, the majority of trans fats will disappear from our food supply.

Monounsaturated and polyunsaturated fats. There are two classes of unsaturated fats. They are both good for you and good for your heart. Foods rich in monounsaturated fatty acids (also called omega-9 fatty acids) include nuts such as macadamias, hazelnuts, pecans, cashews, and peanuts; olive, canola, and soybean oils; olives, soybeans, and avocados.

Polyunsaturated fats are divided further into omega-3 fatty acids and omega-6 fatty acids. Omega-3 fatty acids have gained a lot of attention in recent years because of their role in preventing heart disease. They are essential, meaning your body needs them but cannot make them. They are in salmon, tuna, sardines, mackerel, herring, and other seafood as well as in walnuts, ground flaxseed, and canola and soybean oils. The

American Heart Association recognizes that the omega-3 fatty acids from fish are especially protective of the heart. They recommend the following:

➤ People without coronary heart disease should consume oily fish at least twice weekly and regularly consume walnuts, canola oil, and other plant foods with omega-3 fatty acids.

➤ If you have documented heart disease, talk to your health-care team about getting one gram of omega-3 fatty acids from fish sources each day.

Omega-6 fatty acids are also essential to the diet. They are far more abundant than omega-3 fatty acids and are found in a wide variety of foods, including corn, corn oil, sunflower oil, wheat, chicken, and nuts. At one point, many people, including many health professionals, believed that a high intake of omega-6 fatty acids increased inflammation in the body, thus raising the risk for heart disease and other chronic illnesses. Most experts are no longer concerned about this. In fact, a science advisory from the American Heart Association states that omega-6 fatty acids should make up at least 5–10% of daily calories, which is consistent with current intakes in the United States. Again, your best strategy is to replace saturated and trans fat with any type of unsaturated fat.

Sources of Omega-3 Fatty Acids

➤ Salmon
➤ Herring
➤ Sardines
➤ Rainbow trout
➤ Albacore tuna
➤ Walnuts
➤ Flaxseed, ground
➤ Chia seeds
➤ Canola oil
➤ Soybean oil

Take Action

Cook more with oils and less with butter, stick margarine, lard, shortening, and bacon grease. Identify other ways to replace some saturated fatty acids with monounsaturated or polyunsaturated fatty acids. Especially seek out omega-3 fatty acids, since Americans tend to eat little of these.

Fat Facts

It's not possible to eliminate all saturated fats. We often hear that this food is monounsaturated and that food is saturated, but this is an over-simplification. When we eat fat, we consume a mix of fatty acids: saturated, monounsaturated, and polyunsaturated fatty acids. Even salmon, nuts, and olive oil, which are packed with heart-healthy fats, contain some saturated fatty acids. To eliminate all saturated fats, you would have to eliminate all fat, and that would leave you with very little to eat. For example, olive oil is frequently identified as a monounsaturated fat, but it contains more than that. One tablespoon of olive oil contains:

> ➤ 1.9 g of saturated fatty acids
> ➤ 1.4 g of polyunsaturated fatty acids
> ➤ 9.9 g of monounsaturated fatty acids

Read labels for saturated fats, trans fats, and cholesterol. Limit your intake of each. Eat fish at least twice weekly. Find plenty of delicious fish recipes on the American Diabetes Association's website at diabetes.org/mfa-recipes.

How Different Foods Affect Your Heart

Across the Internet and in popular media, there is a lot of discussion about which foods boost heart health and which foods harm the heart. Sometimes you'll find the same food on both lists, depending on the source or the week. There's no denying that it can be very confusing. Below are discussions of 18 foods or categories of food that patients with diabetes, heart disease, or concerns of general wellness ask about often. Keep in mind that this is just a short list. They are included simply because they are a common source of confusion or interest.

Nuts

Since 2003, the U.S. Food and Drug Administration (FDA) has allowed a qualified health claim on almonds, hazelnuts, peanuts, pecans, pistachios, walnuts, and some pine nuts. It states that evidence suggests (but does not prove) that eating 1.5 ounces of nuts daily as part of a diet low in saturated fat and cholesterol reduces heart-disease risk. To quantify the cardiovascular benefits of nuts, researchers pooled data from several studies. They found that participants who included nuts in their diets experienced an average of 5.1% reduction in total cholesterol and a 7.4% decrease in LDL cholesterol. Individuals with high triglycerides had a

10.2% decline in serum triglyceride levels. Different types of nuts had similar effects, but the effects were dose-related, meaning that the more nuts consumed, the greater were the improvements.

Nuts contain heart-healthy monounsaturated and polyunsaturated fats and so much more; they also give us fiber, vitamins, minerals, plant sterols, antioxidants, and other phytochemicals (plant compounds known to have health-boosting effects). Remember that nuts, like all foods rich in fat, pack a lot of calories in a small amount. Unless you are trying to gain weight, be careful to replace other foods with nuts rather than simply adding them to your diet. Nut butters are also a good option. Look for the presence of partially hydrogenated oils in the ingredients list. If you see this harmful ingredient, put the nut butter back on the shelf and look for a more suitable brand. Often, the all-natural varieties are an ideal choice. The ingredients should be nothing more than nuts and salt.

Flaxseeds and Chia Seeds

Both of these seeds have been dubbed "superfoods." No food deserves such a reputation, because no one food can transform a diet or prevent disease by itself. However, both chia seeds and ground flaxseeds provide ALA, an omega-3 fatty acid. As discussed in the previous chapter, the American Heart Association recommends regularly eating foods that provide ALA, including walnuts, ground flaxseed, chia seeds, and canola oil. You do not need to grind chia seeds to make use of their omega-3 fats, but you do need to grind flaxseeds (or buy them already ground), because the body cannot break them down enough to extract these beneficial fatty acids. Store ground flaxseeds in the refrigerator or freezer to prevent spoilage.

A small amount of ALA is converted within the body to two other omega-3 fatty acids, EPA and DHA. These two are marine-based fatty acids, so we get them when we eat fish. All omega-3 fatty acids have important roles in health; however, research suggests a greater role for EPA and DHA in the prevention of heart disease. See chapter 10 for a discussion about fish and omega-3 fatty acids.

Olive Oil

Olive oil is rich in heart-healthy monounsaturated fatty acids. If you replace butter, bacon grease, or other unhealthy fat with olive oil, you can expect to see improvements in your blood lipids. It appears, how-ever, that olive oil may have additional benefits. When researchers gave two tablespoons of olive oil daily to participants with endothelial dysfunction, the participants exhibited improved endothelial function compared to participants in a control group. Recall from chapter 1 that the endothelium is the thin layer of cells that lines and protects the blood vessel. Olive oil is rich in phytochemicals that may have anti-inflammatory properties and relax blood vessels.

Other Vegetable Oils

Olive oil is not the only heart-healthy oil. When unsaturated fatty acids replace some saturated fatty acids in the diet, total cholesterol and LDL cholesterol levels drop, decreasing cardiovascular risk. Other oils rich in monounsaturated and polyunsaturated fats include canola, corn, peanut, sunflower, and soybean oils.

Caution: Do not simply add olive oil or other oils to your diet unless you need to gain weight. To keep your calories in check, use these oils to replace other fats with these oils.

Tropical Oils

The tropical oils include coconut, palm, and palm kernel oils. These are vegetables oils because they come from plants; however, both the American Heart Association and the Dietary Guidelines Advisory Committee recommend avoiding the tropical oils because their fatty acids are largely saturated.

Avocados

This creamy fruit is rich in heart-healthy monounsaturated fats. Don't let that sway you into eating a whole avocado, however. One-quarter of a medium avocado provides about 65 calories. Slip a few pieces onto a sandwich or into a salad. One way to trim saturated fats from your baked goods is to replace butter with mashed avocado.

Coffee

Grandma may have told you that it stunts your growth. It doesn't. Maybe you've heard that it's bad for your heart. It probably isn't, and it may even be good for your heart. Some studies have linked drinking coffee to a reduced risk of developing type 2 diabetes as well as less risk from dying from coronary artery disease. The caffeine in coffee may, however, temporarily raise your blood pressure. Choose decaffeinated coffee or discuss the use of caffeine with a member of your health-care team. If you drink unfiltered coffee, consider switching to a filtered beverage. Filtering coffee with a paper filter removes cafestol and kahweol, compounds that raise both total and LDL cholesterol. Finally, coffee can be a nutritional blunder if you add syrups, sugar, and cream. Keep your nearly zero-calorie beverage low-calorie by drinking it black, with no-calorie sweeteners, skim milk, or fat-free half-and-half.

Tea

Black, green, oolong, and white teas come from the Camellia sinensis plant. Each of these teas is packed with flavonoids, a class of phytochemical health boosters. Studies suggest that tea drinking is associated with a reduced risk of heart attack and stroke and may help lower blood pressure. Skip the bottled teas, however. They have very little, if any, flavonoids. When making iced tea, brew it double strength and keep it for just a day or two. The older it is, the more the flavonoids break down and lose their disease-fighting potential.

Beans

Beans really are good for the heart, and likely for many reasons. They contain more protein than other vegetables and provide resistant starch, a unique carbohydrate that, when degraded by bacteria in the gut, causes the production of a fatty acid that appears to improve insulin action and lower blood glucose. Rich also in dietary fiber, potassium, magnesium, folate, and a host of phytochemicals, beans are linked to lower blood pressure and reduced risk of heart disease. Eating at least four servings of beans per week is linked to a 22% lower risk of coronary heart disease compared to eating them less than once weekly. A simple way to get beans most days of the week is to open a can of your favorite variety and add a handful to a tossed salad every evening. Drain and rinse canned beans to lower their sodium content by about 40%.

Oats

You may see the following on food labels: "3 grams of soluble fiber daily from oatmeal, in a diet low in saturated fat and cholesterol, may reduce the risk of heart disease." The FDA permits this claim because the fiber in oats acts like a sponge, sopping up cholesterol from your digestive tract and preventing it from entering into your bloodstream. This fiber, called beta-glucan, may help your diabetes as well. It appears to improve insulin action and lower blood glucose. Don't feel that you have to stick to oats all the time. Barley also contains beta-glucan and offers similar health effects. You won't likely find beta-glucan listed on food labels, but do check oat and barley products for soluble fiber content.

Grains

Grains are much maligned, but not rightfully so. In a study of nearly 8,000 women with type 2 diabetes, higher intakes of whole grains, bran, and fiber from cereals were associated with less overall mortality and less death from cardiovascular disease during a 26-year follow up. According to the Dietary Guidelines for Americans, limited evidence suggests that the consumption of whole grains may help prevent type 2 diabetes. Whole grain foods provide fiber, vitamins, minerals, phytochemicals, phytoestrogens, and other compounds, which appear to improve cholesterol levels, lower blood pressure, improve insulin and glucose metabolism, reduce inflammation, and improve endothelial function.

Even refined grains have something to offer. If they have been enriched (and most have been), they provide B vitamins and iron that were stripped away in the processing, along with additional folic acid, which has been instrumental in reducing the number of pregnancies affected by devastating neural tube defects. Unfortunately, however, Americans consume 200% of the recommended amount of refined grains and only 15% of the whole grain target. It is important to replace some servings of refined grains with whole grains. At least half of our grain intake should be whole grains. When buying breads, crackers, cereals, and the like, look carefully at the ingredients list to identify whole grains. If the first ingredient other than water is a whole grain, the product is likely to be mostly or entirely whole grain. Whole grains include the following:

- ❯ Whole wheat
- ❯ Whole rye
- ❯ Oats, oatmeal, rolled oats
- ❯ Whole grain corn
- ❯ Whole grain barley

- ❯ Wild rice
- ❯ Brown rice
- ❯ Millet
- ❯ Popcorn
- ❯ Quinoa

If the label says "made with whole grains," be skeptical. This description tells you little. Without looking more carefully at the label, you cannot know if the product is made with a little or a lot of whole grains. "Enriched wheat flour" is another way of saying "refined flour."

Potatoes

This starchy vegetable also has an undeserved bad reputation. Some people with diabetes fear potatoes and other starchy foods because of their expected effect on blood glucose. The effect on your blood glucose depends on how much potato you eat and what you eat with it, among other factors. You can be confident that when you eat a small potato

---

Hint: Learn How Foods Affect Your Blood Glucose

Though this was discussed in chapter 6, it is worth repeating because there is no better way to learn about the effects of your food choices and portion sizes: Measure your blood glucose right before eating a meal and again 2 hours later. The difference between the two numbers helps you to see how the food you just ate affected your blood glucose. Ideally the difference between the two numbers will be ≤40 or 50 mg/dl. If it is much greater, you may have eaten too much carbohydrate or need additional diabetes medications. Talk to your diabetes educator to fully understand your blood glucose patterns.

Example:

Blood glucose before eating: 104 mg/dl

Blood glucose 2 hours after the first bite: 137 mg/dl

This is acceptable because the change in blood glucose is <40 mg/dl.

The Mystery of the Elevated Cholesterol

Jason loved coffee. Most afternoons, he would take a coffee break at work to visit a café around the corner from his office. He drank it strong and black. Jason's wife surprised him with a French press coffee maker, so he could quickly make coffee at work with little more effort than boiling water in the office microwave. Six months later, Jason had his cholesterol measured. Both he and his health-care provider were confused when the results showed that his total cholesterol had jumped 23 mg/dl and his LDL cholesterol increased by 14 mg/dl since his last blood test a year earlier.

Jason sought advice from a registered dietitian nutritionist (RDN). She recommended that Jason drink only filtered coffee, because unfiltered coffee (French pressed and percolated) is known to increase cholesterol levels. She also suggested that he eat beans a few times each week and add oats and barley to his diet. Jason's cholesterol levels were better than ever at his next doctor's office visit.

(about 5 ounces), you are consuming an affordable source of many needed nutrients, including potassium, magnesium, fiber, vitamin C, and vitamin B6 for about 130 calories and 30 grams of carbohydrate.

Alcohol

Consuming alcohol in moderation is linked with lowered risks of heart disease mortality in people with type 2 diabetes and in the general population. Alcohol may protect the heart by increasing HDL cholesterol. Additionally, the flavonoids and other beneficial compounds in red wine may further benefit the heart by protecting the blood vessels from oxidative damage, though flavonoids are readily available in a variety of fruits, vegetables, and teas. Moderate alcohol intake is also associated with a reduced risk of developing type 2 diabetes, beginning with as little as one-half drink per day. However, alcohol in excess increases the risk of type 2 diabetes and can raise blood pressure, contribute to high triglycerides, produce irregular heartbeats, cause heart failure, and lead to stroke. Both the American Heart Association and the American Diabetes Association recommend that if you don't drink now, you shouldn't start merely to improve heart health. That's because alcohol is linked to too many other chronic diseases and makes you more susceptible to accidents.

You should be aware that alcohol can cause hypoglycemia (low blood glucose), especially among people who take insulin, sulfonylureas, or other drugs that have low blood glucose as a side effect. Hypoglycemia may occur shortly after drinking, or it can happen during the night or the next day, because the liver is unable to supply glucose to the bloodstream. Be sure to eat carbohydrate-containing foods while drinking alcohol. Pretzels, crackers, sandwiches, pasta, and fruit are all good choices. Use extra caution and monitor your blood glucose often when drinking. If you have any question about how your blood glucose is reacting, measure it shortly after drinking, before driving, before going to bed, and even in the middle of the night.

What is moderate drinking? For men, it is having no more than two drinks per day. Because women metabolize alcohol more slowly than men, moderate drinking for women is defined as consuming no more than one drink per day. Often at home and in bars and restaurants, we are served a large glass that is considered more than one drink. The table below shows you how to count a single drink.

What Counts as One Drink?

Alcoholic Beverage	Amount
Beer	12 fluid ounces
	1 bottle or can
Liquor such as bourbon and vodka	1.5 fluid ounces of 80-proof liquor
	1 fluid ounce of 100-proof liquor
Wine	5 fluid ounces

Red Meat

Eating red meat, which includes beef, pork, and lamb, increases the risk of heart disease. For example, in the large Nurses' Health Study that followed women for 26 years, researchers found that women who ate two servings of red meat daily compared to women who ate a half serving per day had a 30% higher risk of developing coronary heart disease. The study further showed that compared to eating one serving of red meat daily, eating one serving of another food in its place had various effects on the risk of developing heart disease.

- Nuts lowered risk by 30%

- Fish lowered risk by 24%

- Poultry lowered risk by 19%

- Low-fat dairy products lowered risk by 13%

Red meat is often rich in saturated fats and cholesterol, which tend to raise LDL cholesterol. But that is probably not the whole story. A study funded partly by the National Institutes of Health (National Heart, Lung, and Blood Institute and the Office of Dietary Supplements) found that gut bacteria metabolize a compound in red meat to a byproduct associated with atherosclerosis. There is still more to learn about the role red meats play in the development of chronic diseases. There are likely additional compounds that contribute to illnesses, so you should limit your intake of beef, pork, and lamb.

Eggs

Eggs are the number one source of cholesterol in the American diet. From a systematic review consisting of 16 published studies, researchers concluded that a single egg per day is not associated with an increased risk of heart disease or stroke in healthy adults. However, they found two important other things of note: First, more than seven eggs weekly is linked with an increased risk of coronary heart disease. Second, among people with type 2 diabetes, egg consumption and high cholesterol intakes are associated with cardiovascular disease risk. Eggs are an inexpensive, convenient source of protein and other nutrients. If you choose to eat eggs, limit your intake of yolks (the source of the cholesterol) and continue to monitor your intake of other sources of cholesterol and saturated and trans fatty acids. See pages 56 and 61 for a list of common sources of saturated fats and dietary cholesterol.

Soy

This is one area where research is inconsistent, though it appears that consuming soy may slightly reduce your LDL and total cholesterol levels. Soy is additionally beneficial if you eat it in place of meats high in saturated fat and cholesterol, such as fried chicken, sausage, and steaks. Among other nutrients, soy provides fiber, omega-3 fatty acids, potassium, and magnesium. Some people have concerns that soy increases the risk of certain cancers. According to the American Institute for Cancer Research, you can put those fears to rest. In fact, soy may even reduce cancer risk.

Not sure what to do with soy? Edamame beans (green soybeans) are available frozen, either shelled or in their pods. They cook quickly in boiling water, and you can eat them plain or added to stir fries, soups, stews, and rice dishes. Choose firm or extra-firm tofu for grilling and soft tofu for smoothies, lasagna, or other casseroles. Many supermarkets also carry tempeh, which is made from cooked and fermented soybeans. Grill a slice for a sandwich.

Chocolate

There's good news here. A number of studies suggest that dark chocolate and cocoa are associated with health benefits related to the heart. Both of these treats are rich sources of flavonoids, and this may be the reason for the observed benefits. Studies suggest that dark chocolate and cocoa have positive effects on blood pressure, HDL cholesterol, oxidation of LDL cholesterol, markers of inflammation, and more. The bad news here is that it is very easy to overdo it. An ounce of chocolate has about 150 calories, similar to the amount in a can of soda. Replace less healthful treats like pastries with dark chocolate to reap its rewards. But do limit yourself to a serving no larger than about an ounce.

Depending on the manufacturer's processing methods, dark chocolate may retain most of its flavonoids or lose most of them. There's no guarantee that a particular chocolate is rich in flavonoids, but dark chocolate supplies more than milk chocolate. When buying cocoa powder, choose one that has not been treated with alkali, also known as Dutch processing, to get the most flavonoids.

Plant Stanols and Sterols

According to the National Cholesterol Education Program (NCEP) of the National Heart, Lung, and Blood Institute, consuming 2 grams of plant stanols and sterols daily can lower LDL cholesterol by as much as 15%. Plant stanols and sterols are the vegetable version of cholesterol, but they are helpful to the heart, not harmful. They are present in small amounts in many foods, including nuts and seeds, soybean and canola oils, and beans. Because they occur in such minute amounts, it's not possible to consume 2 grams of plant stanols and sterols without taking some type of fortified food or supplement. The FDA allows a health claim on foods with added plant stanols and sterols indicating that if eaten twice daily with meals, in the proper amount and with a diet low in saturated fat and cholesterol, they may lower the risk of heart disease. Manufacturers have added these beneficial compounds to some brands of milk, margarine, soymilk, cheese, orange juice, bread, baked goods, and other products. You must substitute these foods for others instead of simply adding them to your diet. Otherwise, you will gain weight. Talk to a registered dietitian nutritionist (RD or RDN) or your health-care provider for more information about the best way to use these foods, and discuss using supplements.

Take Action

Review the foods in this chapter when making your grocery list.

The Impact of Weight

As you saw in chapter 4, being overweight increases your risk for many health problems, including type 2 diabetes and heart disease. Additionally, excess body fat makes it more difficult to control blood pressure, cholesterol, and blood glucose levels. If you are overweight, losing even a few pounds can have profound health benefits.

> One study found that losing 10 pounds was effective in controlling stage 1 high blood pressure.

> Moderate weight loss can improve insulin resistance.

> During the 3-year landmark Diabetes Prevention Program (DPP), adults at high risk for type 2 diabetes reduced their risk of developing the disease by 58% by aiming to lose 7% of their body weight (14 pounds if starting at 200 pounds) and exercising for 150 minutes per week. Even 10 years after the start of the study, these lifestyle interventions had lowered the risk of developing type 2 diabetes by 34%.

> Further analysis of the DPP found that the same lifestyle interventions improved blood pressure, triglyceride, and HDL cholesterol levels as well as measures of inflammation.

- Women with urinary incontinence who lost on average 8% of their body weight (16 pounds if starting at 200 pounds) cut their frequency of incontinence in half.

- Among people with type 2 diabetes, weight loss shortly after diagnosis has both an initial health benefit and long-term benefits on blood pressure and blood glucose control, even if a portion of the lost weight is regained.

- Moderate weight loss improves fertility, pain from osteoarthritis, and much more.

Set a Weight Loss Goal

So you see, you do not need to lose gobs of weight to improve your health. Start with a goal of losing 5–10% of your starting weight. Once you get there, decide if you want to lose more. If so, make your next weight loss goal 5–10% of your new weight. Periodically checking your waist circumference and your BMI can guide your decision about losing any more weight. Remember from chapter 4 that these are not perfect tools to assess body fatness. If you are unsure if you should lose weight, speak with a member of your health-care team. Often, a change in diet and a lower weight will require a change in medications to prevent hypoglycemia, low blood pressure, and other problems.

Your Weight (pounds)	5–10% (pounds)	New Goal Weight (pounds)
120	6–12	108–114
140	7–14	126–133
160	8–16	144–152
180	9–18	162–171
200	10–20	180–190
220	11–22	198–209
240	12–24	216–228
260	13–26	234–247
280	14–28	252–266
300	15–30	270–285
320	16–32	288–304
340	17–34	306–323

Additional Weight Loss Resources

This chapter can get you started on your weight loss plan, but many people will need more help than a single chapter can provide. For individualized help, ask your health-care provider for a referral to a registered dietitian nutritionist. You can find one in your area by visiting the website of the Academy of Nutrition and Dietetics (AND) at eatright.org. The book *Diabetes Weight Loss Week by Week* (American Diabetes Association) will also teach you much of what you need to know. Additionally, you will find weight loss information on the websites of the American Diabetes Association (diabetes.org), the American Heart Association (heart.org), the USDA MyPlate (myplate.gov), and the Centers for Disease Control and Prevention (cdc.gov).

Understand the Calorie Balance Equation

There is no magic plan. There are no foods or pills that melt fat from your thighs or midsection. You do not need to follow a long list of diet rules, and you do not need to give up your favorite foods entirely. You do, however, need to understand that any diet that helps you to lose weight does so because you consume fewer calories than your body burns. This doesn't mean that you have to count calories to lose weight, but it does mean that you will need to change your diet to consume fewer calories, increase your physical activity to burn more calories, or, preferably, both. Chapter 14 is devoted to physical activity.

You should also understand that there is no one best weight-loss diet. Many people lose weight and stay thin by eating a very high carbohydrate, moderate protein vegan diet. Others lose weight with a plan much lower in carbohydrate and higher in protein. Similarly, dieters can lose weight consuming varying amounts of fat. Even without counting calories, however, every successful dieter loses weight because calories consumed are less than calories burned, regardless of the percentage of calories that come from carbohydrate, protein, and fat.

- ❯ Weight maintenance: calories eaten = calories burned
- ❯ Weight loss: calories eaten < calories burned
- ❯ Weight gain: calories eaten > calories burned

Your best diet will be one that you can live with long term, not just for several days, weeks, or months. It will include the foods you enjoy in reasonable quantities, and it will not restrict the foods you need for optimal health. Weight loss cannot be the only goal. Your best diet will also balance enjoyment and good health.

Calorie goal. According to the 2010 Dietary Guidelines for Americans, most women need between 1,600 and 2,400 calories per day to maintain their weight, and men require between 2,000 and 3,000 calories daily for weight maintenance. Cut about 200–600 calories each day to lose weight at a healthful rate. These are broad ranges and may still not cover every man or woman. You can get a better estimate of your calories needs at ChooseMyPlate.gov. There you will enter your age, weight, and activity level to get an estimate of your calorie needs. Again, it's still an estimate, but it is a good starting point. By having a daily calorie goal, you can use food labels and calorie-counting books, apps, and websites to see how a specific food fits into your day. For example, you can ask yourself how a large, plain bagel at 320 calories fits into your 1,600-calorie meal plan. You may then decide to eat only half of the bagel or to eat an English muffin at 140 calories instead.

Eat filling foods. If you are constantly hungry while trimming calories, you will likely give up your weight loss plan and go back to previous eating habits. That's why a smart plan is much more than simply "eating less." In fact, successful dieters often report that they eat more. Indeed, they may have stopped skipping meals and started eating foods that are more filling, take longer to eat, and are more satisfying. These are water-rich and fiber-rich foods such as fruits, vegetables, and broth-based soups. While these dieters are eating more food, they are also eating fewer calories. Research shows us that increasing our intake of lower-calorie foods helps us to eat less of the higher-calorie foods. The following table shows you how foods of equal calories vary in volume. Typically, foods of higher volume are more filling.

Food Providing Approximately 100 Calories

Cheddar cheese, 1-ounce slice	Cherry tomatoes, 33
Jelly donut, 1/3 donut	Apple slices, 1 3/4 cups
Popcorn chicken, 4 1/2 pieces	Blueberries, 1 1/4 cups
Broccoli spears, cooked, 2 cups	Chicken & vegetable soup, 1 1/4 cups

Source: USDA Nutrient Data Laboratory

These books will teach you more about this concept, known as energy density or calorie density.

> *The Ultimate Volumetrics Diet* by Barbara Rolls, PhD with Mindy Hermann, RD

> *The Volumetrics Eating Plan* by Barbara Rolls, PhD

Try to eat fruits and vegetables with every meal and snack to boost nutrition and lower your overall calorie intake. For example, at breakfast decrease your usual amount of cereal and add a large serving of fresh berries. Instead of eating two plain scrambled eggs, have just one with sautéed mushrooms and bell peppers. At lunch, stuff your sandwich with more veggies than meat and cheese. When making pasta salad or rice pilaf, add more vegetables than usual. Shrink your usual meat and starch portions on your dinner plate to make room for double vegetable portions or a low-calorie tossed salad, or start your meal with a cup of vegetable soup.

Trim high-calorie foods. Foods with a lot of fat or added sugars tend to be high-calorie. You probably already know that cheesecake, brownies, and fast food burgers and milkshakes are calorie-dense. But do you know how high? Look up some of your favorite foods in a calorie-counting book, at MyFoodAdvisor.com, or at SuperTracker.usda.gov. You have several options if a favorite food is too high to fit into your diet on a regular basis.

> Eat it rarely.

> Eat a smaller portion. For example, split a slice of cheesecake with two other people, or prepare miniature cheesecakes.

> Find a substitute. Unsweetened applesauce has about half the calories of sweetened applesauce. Nonfat frozen yogurt has fewer calories than premium ice cream.

> Find an alternative cooking method. Baked chicken with the skin removed can substitute for baked or fried chicken with the skin eaten.

Keep making small changes like these, and you will see results over time. Consistency is key.

Drinks count. Coffee with cream and sugar in the morning, a sports drink after aerobics class, sweetened tea with lunch, and a cocktail or soda with dinner add up to several hundred calories by the end of the day. The problem is this: It's so easy to overdo caloric beverages because they just don't feel like they could provide so many calories. Switch a few drinks each day to calorie-free water or unsweetened tea or coffee, and you will save quite a bit of calories over several weeks. Below are the calorie counts for several common beverages.

Beverage	Calories
Café latte, made with whole milk, no sugar, 16 ounces	220
Cola, 12-ounce can	152
Sweetened iced tea, 12 ounces	128
Fruit punch, 12-ounces	175
Lemonade, 8 ounces	99
Sports drink, 8 ounces	63
Wine, red, 5 ounces	125
Beer, 12-ounce can	153

Sources: USDA Nutrient Data Laboratory and Starbucks.com

Portion sense. There is no denying that portions sizes in restaurants and in single-serve bags of chips and cookies have expanded over recent decades. These large portions have spilled into the home, too. Research shows that we unintentionally consume more when we have more in front of us, making it harder to control our weight. Reining in portions can help us rein in calories. Try some of these portion control strategies.

> Minimize second helpings, by serving food from the kitchen instead of serving at the table. The exception is for low-calorie vegetables and salads. Leave these on the table to encourage second helpings.

> Eat only from a dish. Put a measured serving in a bowl or on a plate. It's hard to know how much you're eating when you dig into a box or bag.

> Pre-portion crackers, chips, cookies, and other treats into individual servings.

- Use portion control dishes. A quick search on the Internet will show you many options.

- Buy treats like ice cream in individual servings such as bars and sandwiches, or ask someone else to scoop your serving.

- Weigh and measure foods for a few days to get a sense of the amount of food you eat.

- Stretch out your meals. Sip water, put your fork down between bites, and savor every bite.

Eating out. Restaurant meals bring a unique set of concerns. The portions are large, and it's hard to know what has been cooked in spoonfuls of butter or lard and what is sweetened with excessive amounts of sugar. Asking a lot of questions is your best way to learn how a food is prepared. Here are more tips to help you enjoy a restaurant meal without breaking the calorie bank.

- Preview the menu online or call ahead to learn about the menu.

- Share a meal with a dining companion or bring home leftovers for lunch. No super-sizing allowed.

- Ask the waiter not to bring bread, muffins, or tortilla chips. If others at the table want them, push them to the far side of the table.

- Start your meal with a salad or broth-based soup. Order double vegetables.

- Treat yourself to no more than one splurge food. Do you want drinks, bread, dessert, or a fried appetizer? Commit to just one.

- Use caution with foods marked "low-carb." Often these are the menu items highest in saturated fat and calories.

- Ask for sauces and dressings on the side.

- Avoid these restaurant terms that are code for high-fat or high-calorie:
  - Au gratin, crispy, buttered, creamed, Alfredo, rich, coated, basted, deep-fried.

To identify national and local restaurants that serve healthful meals, visit Healthy Dining Finder at HealthyDiningFinder.com. Check out these two books as well.

> *Guide to Healthy Restaurant Eating*, 4th edition, by Hope S. Warshaw, MMSc, RD, CDE (American Diabetes Association, 2009)

> *Eat Out Healthy* by Joanne V. Lichten, PhD, RD (Nutrifit Publishing, 2011)

Keep a Record

Food records work. Research studies prove that people who record their food intake lose more weight than people who do not. You can jot down your food intake in a notebook, a computer spreadsheet, or even on scrap paper. The key is to be honest and record everything. Write down what you eat as you go through your day instead of reporting back at the end of the day or the end of the week. Review your food intake daily. Ask yourself what can you learn from this and how can you do better. It's not enough to write it down and pay no attention to it later.

Keep in mind that weight management is hard. Expect to work hard at it and to have both successes and failures. Consistency will make a difference in the long run. If you need help, ask for it.

Should You Consider Weight Loss Surgery?

Weight loss surgery, also called bariatric surgery, is for the severely overweight only. There are various types of weight loss surgery, and the amount of weight you can expect to lose varies with the type. Many people lose one-third of their starting bodyweight or more. Some procedures result in an average weight loss of about 15% of starting weight. The remission rates for type 2 diabetes also vary and may range from less than 50% to about 95%. Weight loss surgery is not for everyone. It is not without risks, so the risks and benefits must be carefully weighed.

Red Flags of Weight Loss Fads

If it sounds too good to be true, it probably is. Steer clear of any questionable program. Watch out for programs doing or claiming any of the following:

> You can eat all you want and lose weight without exercise.
> The program or product works for everyone. (Actually, diets should be individualized to the dieter's preferences and medical history.)
> Calories don't count. (You know that they do count!)
> Eliminates a large list of foods or whole food groups.
> Requires odd food combinations or has a long list of diet rules.
> You can drop 15 pounds in one week. (Healthful weight loss is about 1–2 pounds per week, perhaps a little more initially.)
> Weight loss is permanent. (Maintaining lower weight requires lifestyle changes.)
> Bases claims on before and after photos and testimonials from dieters. (Nutrition is a science, so be skeptical if the only "proof" is someone's emotional story and photo.)
> Uses words like "breakthrough," "secret formula," and "miraculous."
> Requires you to commit a large sum of money or tells you that you must sign up now before there is a price increase.

Take Action

Check with your health-care provider before significantly changing your diet. If you need to lose weight, choose an initial weight loss goal that is 5–10% of your current weight. Determine your approximate calorie needs, and identify a few places in your diet to reduce your calorie intake. Record your food intake daily.

How to Change Your Diet

Several of the last chapters reviewed food and diet and have offered suggestions for foods to eat and those to avoid. This chapter shows you some ways in which you can make the recommended changes at home and when eating away from home.

Keep in mind that you should not change everything at once if it means that you will be able to stick to your new eating plan for only a few weeks or months. It's far better to focus on those dietary changes that are most important to you. Integrate them fully into your life and then make additional changes. The pace is up to you. Move as quickly or as slowly as is reasonable, understanding that everyone will progress at a different pace and will have different priorities.

If, for example, you eat fried foods several times a week, you might set a goal of eating them only once per week. If, on the other hand, you rarely eat fried foods, but your blood pressure is out of control, you may want to start with cutting back on salt and eating more fruits and vegetables, since they are rich in blood pressure–friendly potassium.

Once you recognize your dietary weaknesses and feel that it's time to make a change, pick a very specific behavioral goal. It should be so clear that you know exactly how to proceed. For example, *to eat better* or *to eat smaller portions* is very vague. A goal to eat fruits and/or vegetables at every meal is specific and clear. So is a goal to limit starchy foods to 1 cup or two slices of bread at each meal. Review your current diet, and get started with one or a handful of dietary improvements.

The following food swaps and menu revisions will show you several ways to start eating better.

Make the Swap in Cooking and Baking

Instead of This	Try This	Your Reward
Butter in baking	3 Tbsp olive or canola oil to replace 4 Tbsp butter	Less unhealthy fats; more healthy fats
Butter in cooking	Olive, canola, or other cooking oils	Less unhealthy fats; more healthy fats
Butter on toast	Peanut butter, almond butter, or other nut butter	Less unhealthy fats; more healthy fats, protein, vitamins, minerals, fiber, phytochemicals
Cheese on a sandwich	Reduced-fat cheese	Less unhealthy fats and calories
	Avocado	Less unhealthy fats; more healthy fats, fiber, and phytochemicals, and a different array of vitamins and minerals
Egg	2 egg whites	Less saturated fat, cholesterol, calories
Cream sauce on pasta	Wine sauce or garlic and olive oil sauce	Less unhealthy fats; more healthy fats
	Tomato sauce	Less unhealthy fats; more vitamins, minerals, fiber, phytochemicals
Blue cheese or ranch dressing	Vinaigrette or oil and vinegar dressing	Less unhealthy fats; more healthy fats
	Avocado dressing	Less unhealthy fats; more healthy fats, fiber, phytochemicals
Onion or cheese dip	Hummus	Less unhealthy fats; more healthy fats, protein, fiber, phytochemicals

Instead of This	Try This	Your Reward
Bread crumbs	Rolled oats or crushed bran cereal	Less refined flour; more vitamins, minerals, fiber, phytochemicals
	Chopped walnuts or other nuts	Less refined flour; more healthy fats, vitamins, minerals, fiber, phytochemicals
White flour	White whole wheat flour	More vitamins, minerals, fiber
	Whole wheat flour	More vitamins, minerals, fiber, phytochemicals
Garlic salt	Fresh garlic or garlic powder	Less sodium
Lemon pepper	Sodium-free lemon pepper	Less sodium

Make the Swap in the Supermarket

Instead of This	Try This	Your Reward
Whole milk	1% or nonfat milk	Less unhealthy fats and calories
Bottled tea, sweetened	Tea bags	Less added sugars, no calories; more flavonoid phytochemicals
Canned fruit with added sugar	Canned fruit without added sugar	Less calories and added sugars
	Fresh fruit	Less calories and added sugars; sometimes more fiber and other nutrients
Fruit-on-the-bottom yogurt	Nonfat or low-fat Greek yogurt and fresh fruit	Less calories and added sugars; more vitamins, minerals, fiber, phytochemicals
Large bagel	English muffin or small bagel	Less calories and carbohydrates by about half
Snack crackers	Almonds, peanuts, walnuts, or other nuts	No refined grains, less carbohydrates; more healthy fats, vitamins, minerals, fiber, phytochemicals
Instant flavored oatmeal	Instant plain oatmeal	Less calories and added sugars
Soy sauce	Low-sodium soy sauce	Less sodium

Instead of This	Try This	Your Reward
Spaghetti	Whole wheat spaghetti Combination white/whole wheat spaghetti	Less refined flour; more fiber, phytochemicals
White rice	Brown rice, wild rice, barley, quinoa	More vitamins, minerals, fiber, phytochemicals
Frozen dinner	Lower-sodium, lower-fat frozen meal such as Healthy Choice	Depending on the meal chosen: less calories, sodium, unhealthy fats

Make the Swap When Eating Out

Instead of This	Try This	Your Reward
Iced tea with sugar	Unsweetened tea with lemon	Less calories and added sugars
Café latte, regular	Café latte, nonfat	Less calories and unhealthy fats
New England clam chowder	Manhattan clam chowder	Less calories and unhealthy fats
Thick crust pepperoni pizza	Thin crust veggie pizza	Less calories, unhealthy fats, carbohydrates
Large burger and fries	Small burger and fries with a side salad	Less calories, unhealthy fats, carbohydrates; more vitamins, minerals, phytochemicals
10-ounce steak	4-ounce steak	Less calories and unhealthy fats
Egg roll	Steamed dumplings	Less calories and unhealthy fats
Fried chicken	Rotisserie chicken without skin	Less calories and unhealthy fats
Bacon	Canadian bacon	Less calories and unhealthy fats
Omelet	Egg white omelet	Less unhealthy fats, cholesterol, calories

The following menus offer additional suggestions to make a mediocre diet better and then even better than that. The column labeled *Even Better* isn't perfect. You can find ways to make it better still. There is no one perfect diet, so there are many paths you can follow to a healthier plate. Use these menus as inspiration to come up with your own ways to make your diet better.

	Typical Diet	Better	Even Better
Breakfast	Pastry 2 fried eggs 8 ounces orange juice Coffee with sugar and cream	Toast with peanut butter 1 scrambled egg, cooked in canola oil 1% milk 4 ounces orange juice Coffee with sugar and 1% milk	Whole wheat toast with peanut butter Vegetable omelet with 1 whole egg and additional egg whites, cooked in canola oil 1% milk Small orange Coffee with 1% milk, artificial sweetener, optional
Lunch	Broccoli cheese soup Roast beef sandwich with mustard and mayonnaise Sweetened iced tea	Lentil soup Turkey sandwich on whole wheat bread with mustard, light mayonnaise, lettuce, tomato, bell peppers Unsweetened iced tea	Lentil soup with nonfat Greek yogurt Mixed green salad with olive oil–based vinaigrette Mixed berries Unsweetened iced tea
Dinner	10-ounce steak Iceberg lettuce wedge with blue cheese dressing White rice with butter Soda	5-ounce steak Iceberg lettuce wedge with reduced-fat dressing Brown rice with soft spread 1% milk	4 ounces baked salmon with mango-tomato salsa Spinach sautéed in olive oil Barley, brown rice, or quinoa pilaf 1% milk
Snacks	Chips Crackers and cheese	1/4 cup almonds and walnuts Whole grain crackers and reduced-fat cheese	1/4 cup almonds and walnuts Low-fat cottage cheese with diced tomatoes and fresh basil

Take Action

Set one to five very specific behavioral goals. Decide what you will do to improve your diet and exactly how you will do it.

The Power of Exercise

Have you heard that exercise is the greatest medicine? Health professionals often say this, because being physically active helps prevent and treat so many health concerns and illnesses. Here's what exercise can do for you:

> Boost mood

> Offer you a sense of accomplishment

> Lower your blood pressure

> Improve insulin action and blood glucose control

> Aid weight loss

> Enhance your immune system

> Improve circulation

> Increase HDL cholesterol

> Help manage stress

> Prevent bone loss

> Improve sleep

> Build muscle strength

Additionally, regular exercise helps prevent type 2 diabetes, heart disease, stroke, osteoporosis, overweight and obesity, and several types of cancer. Unfortunately, only 58% of adults in the United States are physically active, which is defined as doing 30 minutes of moderate or vigorous activity three times weekly. Even worse is that only 39% of adults with diabetes are physically active.

How Much Should You Exercise?

Even a single bout of exercise can improve blood glucose levels for 2–72 hours after exercise. The greatest benefits, of course, occur with regular exercise, and this is true even without weight loss. Any amount of exercise is better than none. If you have just 10 minutes, exercise for 10 minutes. Even if you have only 8, go for it. Though the proper exercise prescription will depend on your preferences, medications, health conditions, blood glucose control, risk for hypoglycemia, and more, the American Diabetes Association has general guidelines.

> If able, adults with diabetes should engage in at least 150 minutes of moderate-intensity aerobic activity each week, over at least 3 days, and without more than 2 days in a row without exercise.

> If able, adults should also engage in resistance exercises on nonconsecutive days at least twice weekly, but preferably three times per week.

Check with your health-care provider before starting an exercise program. Even most people with existing heart disease and other diabetes complications can exercise safely, though your health-care provider may want to run additional tests to determine the types of exercise that are safest for you.

Components of an Exercise Plan

A complete exercise program includes four types of exercise.

Aerobic exercise. This is sometimes called cardiorespiratory or cardiovascular exercise. It is continuous exercise that uses large muscle groups and causes your heart to beat faster and for you to breathe heavily. Becoming aerobically fit allows your heart, lungs, and blood vessels to efficiently transport oxygen throughout your body. Aerobic activities include walking, jogging, running, biking, swimming, dancing, jumping rope, raking leaves, cross-country skiing, rollerblading, and so much more. Aerobic exercise helps to control weight and improves insulin action.

Resistance exercise. Lifting weights, using elastic bands, and performing sit-ups and push-ups are examples of resistance exercises. These types of exercises increase muscular strength (how much your muscles can do or lift) and muscular endurance (how long your muscles can do it). They can also increase bone mass and bone strength, help you maintain independence in activities of daily living as you age, and reduce your risk of injury. Regular resistance training improves insulin sensitivity at least as well as aerobic exercise. And the combination of aerobic training and resistance training is greater than either of the two alone.

Flexibility exercises. Stretching exercises will help you maintain or improve the range of motion of your joints. Joint flexibility tends to decrease with age, but regular flexibility exercises can improve your range of motion no matter how old you are. Yoga and tai chi include basic stretching movements. Follow these guidelines for safe and productive stretching:

> Stretch warm muscles to reduce the risk of injury. Either stretch after performing other exercises when your muscles have greater blood flow, or warm up with light walking or other movement for at least 5 minutes.

> Avoid bouncing during stretching.

> At least two to three times weekly, stretch each of these major muscle groups: neck, shoulders, lower back, hips, thighs, and calves.

> Hold a stretch for 15–30 seconds. Repeat the exercise until you have stretched the muscle for a total of 60 seconds.

Balance exercise. Improving your balance can be as simple as practicing standing on one leg and performing similar exercises several times per week. Some people enjoy and benefit from exercise games such as the Wii Fit that provide balance games. Among the elderly, balance training decreases the risk for falls. This is especially important for individuals with peripheral neuropathy (nerve damage to the peripheral nervous system, often in the feet and legs), because they are especially likely to fall.

Getting Started

If you are inactive, simply adding movement into your day offers great benefits. In fact, even people who regularly exercise for an hour daily need to avoid long periods of inactivity to further reduce their risk for metabolic syndrome and other health problems. Taking several exercise breaks of 1–5 minutes each during the day is beneficial. You can do this in a structured way such as walking or stretching for a couple minutes every hour. Or you can do this in an unstructured manner, such as using the restroom far from you, parking far away in the parking lot, getting off the bus or subway one stop early, standing instead of sitting, walking while talking on the phone, folding laundry, changing TV channels without using the remote control, and more.

Many people enjoy using a pedometer for motivation. A basic pedometer is nothing more than a step counter, and this is all you really need. Fancy models may estimate your distance or calories expended. They may have 7-day memories or connect to your computers and create graphs of your progress. If you enjoy gadgets, you might like these fancier models. If not, stick to a simple step counter. Just be certain that it is a good model that counts your steps accurately. A few accurate brands include Omron, Accusplit, and Yamax.

> ➤ To check the accuracy of your pedometer, clip it to your waistband above the center of your knee, and set it to zero. A good pedometer will measure steps only, and will not count every twist and turn as a step. Wiggle around a bit to see how yours does. Next, with your pedometer still set at zero, walk exactly 100 steps. If your pedometer registers between 90 and 110 steps, it is accurate enough. If it appears inaccurate or if your pants roll down at the waistband or are very loose, turn the pedometer inward so it faces your body, or try it on the small of your back. If none of these positions provide for accurate counting, you should try a different brand of pedometer.

> ➤ Use a safety strap with your pedometer to prevent losing it should it fall off.

> ➤ Wear your pedometer all day for several days to determine your average number of steps. Then set a goal to increase your average

number of steps by 500–2,000 steps daily. A typical long-term goal is 10,000 steps per day.

➤ Each day, reset your pedometer to zero. Strap it on and start moving.

FITT Goals for Better Fitness

Improving your fitness level will take time, energy, and a plan. Start your plan by writing a specific goal using the FITT principle.

F: Frequency: How often will you do a particular exercise?

I: Intensity: How vigorously will you exercise?

T: Time: How many minutes will you perform the exercise?

T: Type: What type of exercise will you do?

You can apply the FITT principle to each of the four components of a fitness plan. To build your aerobic fitness with walking, your FITT goal might look like this:

F: at least 4 times per week

I: at a moderate pace (you can hold a conversation)

T: for at least 10 minutes

T: walking

As your fitness level improves, you can increase the frequency, intensity, or time. Eventually, you can increase all three. Use the FITT principle to plan each component of your fitness program. If you need guidance, schedule an appointment with a member of your health-care team or ask for recommendations to work with a certified personal trainer who has experience working with people similar to you in age and health status.

Safety Precautions

Though the benefits of being physically active nearly always outweigh the health risks, you must still exercise with safety in mind. Some people will have exercise restrictions because of a health condition (see Exercise Limitations for People with Complications of Diabetes below), but everyone with diabetes must follow basic safety precautions.

> Monitor your blood glucose before and after activity to learn how various exercises and levels of intensity affect you. Understand that if you take insulin or a medication that causes your pancreas to produce more insulin, exercise may cause your blood glucose to drop too low for as much as a full day after exercising. Exercise with a partner until you have learned how your blood glucose responds to exercise.

> If you take a medication that can cause hypoglycemia and your blood glucose is <100 mg/dl before exercising, you may need a snack of 20–30 grams of carbohydrate prior to exercising. See the "Snacking Before and After Exercise" section below.

> Do not exercise if your blood glucose is >250 mg/dl and you have ketones in your urine or blood.

> If you are at risk for hypoglycemia, carry glucose tablets, glucose gels, or another source of rapidly absorbed carbohydrate. Carry your blood glucose meter with you as well. See pages 33–34 for the "Rule of 15" to treat hypoglycemia.

> If necessary, use sports gels, drinks, and bars during physical activity.

> If you take insulin, ask your health-care provider about reducing your dose before exercising. Avoid exercising when the insulin peaks (the time when it is working at its strongest).

> Wear some form of diabetes identification.

> Avoid exercising in extreme temperatures. It's good to have both indoor and outdoor exercise options.

> Wear properly fitted shoes and clean socks made of material that draws the sweat away from your feet.

> Examine your feet daily and before and after exercise. Look for red spots, blisters, and sores. Tend to them immediately.

> Stop exercising if you experience pain, lightheadedness, or short-ness of breath.

Exercise Limitations for People with Complications of Diabetes

If you have complications or other health problems, your health-care provider may restrict certain activities and encourage others. Below are general guidelines, but you must find out what is best for you.

Health Condition	General Recommendations
Retinopathy (eye disease)	If you have proliferative retinopathy or severe nonproliferative retinopathy, you may be advised to avoid high-intensity or high-impact exercises, heavy lifting, holding your breath, and placing your head below the level of your heart. Low-impact exercises like walking and stationary biking are usually okay. There are generally no restrictions for mild nonproliferative retinopathy.
Peripheral neuropathy in the feet and legs	If you have a foot ulcer or an open sore, avoid walking, dancing, and other weight-bearing activities. It's okay to engage in moderate weight-bearing activities if you do not have sores. Cycling, swimming, and chair exercises are good activity choices.
Autonomic neuropathy	This type of nerve damage may affect the heart, lungs, stomach, intestines, bladder, or genitals. You may be advised to monitor your heart rate, avoid exercising in extreme heat or cold, and avoid high-intensity activities. Your health-care provider may want to perform tests before giving you approval to exercise.
Heart disease	You may be advised to monitor your heart rate, avoid exercising in extreme heat or cold, and avoid high-intensity activities. Walking and low-intensity resistance exercises are frequently okay.

Snacking Before and After Exercise

Not everyone needs a snack before exercise or even after exercise. For some people, the only thing snacking does is provide extra calories, making weight management more difficult, or extra carbohydrates, making blood glucose management more difficult. However, if you take insulin or another medication that has hypoglycemia as a side effect, you may need a pre- or postexercise snack or both to keep your blood glucose from dropping too low. If you use insulin, you may need a snack of 10–30 grams of carbohydrate for every 30–45 minutes of moderate physical activity. If you are at risk for low blood glucose, eating a carbohydrate-containing snack within 30 minutes to 2 hours after exercising may help prevent hypoglycemia. You may need another carbohydrate-containing snack before bed to prevent later-onset hypoglycemia in the middle of the night. Monitoring your blood glucose often will help you learn how various types and intensities of exercise affect you.

Good choices for pre-exercise snacks include foods with both carbohydrate and protein.

➤ Half a turkey sandwich

➤ Greek yogurt and fruit

➤ Apple and cheese stick

➤ Low-fat cottage cheese with crackers or fruit

Good choices for postexercise snacks include foods with a mix of carbohydrates, protein, and fat.

➤ Chocolate milk

➤ Whole milk

➤ Apples slice with peanut butter and a cheese stick

➤ Slice of veggie pizza

Blood Glucose Goals During Physical Activity

Ask your health-care provider what is best for you. As a general guideline, if you use insulin, aim to keep your blood glucose level >110 mg/dl during physical activity. If you use other diabetes medications that may cause low blood glucose, aim for >90 mg/dl during exercise. Sports bars, gels, and drinks may be good food choices during exercise. If the medications you take to manage your blood glucose do not have hypoglycemia as a side effect, you should not be concerned about a minimum blood glucose level.

Overcoming Barriers to Exercise

I'm too tired. I'm too busy. I get too sweaty. The weather is bad. These are all common reasons for not being physically active. Sometimes they are true barriers that need solutions. Other times, they are simply excuses for not exercising. Give your situation an honest appraisal. Are these simply excuses? If so, vow now to stop making excuses. If you have real barriers to exercise, start looking for solutions. Most likely, there is more than one good solution.

Barrier: Bad weather
Solutions: Find both an indoor and outdoor activity that you enjoy. Buy appropriate exercise clothing for the weather. Carry a water bottle with you.

Barrier: Too busy
Solutions: Get up 20 minutes early each day for a 15-minute walk. Delegate household chores or errands to others to free up time. Instead of scheduling a lunch date, meet friends for a walk, a tennis game, or a bike ride. Break up exercise into three 10-minute bouts instead of one 30-minute bout. Turn on your favorite music and dance for 10 minutes. Recognize that any exercise is better than none. Do household chores such as vacuuming and dusting in a vigorous way.

Barrier: Too tired
Solutions: Schedule your bedtime and stick to it. Exercise early in the day or at lunchtime. Take a 10-minute walk just before leaving work for the day or stop at the gym before heading home. Consider that exercise boosts energy. Find an energizing activity like dancing. Use a pedometer and aim for just a small increase such as 500 additional steps.

Barrier: Exercise is boring
Solutions: Experiment with new activities such as line dancing, inline skating, surfing, tennis, spin class, yoga, tai chi, water aerobics, or Zumba. Exercise with a friend.

Take Action

Before starting an exercise program, check in with your health-care provider to see if you need a medical work-up. Ask if you have exercise limitations and discuss blood glucose control during and after physical activity. Once you have the go-ahead, pick an activity and decide when you will exercise. Identify any barriers to exercise and their possible solutions.

Resources to Help with Diet and Exercise

Often the primary health-care provider or a nurse in the same office can offer basic information about diet and exercise. Usually, however, when it comes to individualized advice and goal setting, you will need to make appointments with other experts. A registered dietitian (RD or RDN) is the food and nutrition expert. You can get expert fitness advice from an exercise physiologist, physical therapist, or a certified personal trainer.

Food and Nutrition Support and Advice

Ask your health-care provider for a referral to a registered dietitian for medical nutrition therapy. Ideally, the registered dietitian will also be a certified diabetes educator (CDE). A registered dietitian (RD, also known as an RDN for "registered dietitian nutritionist") has training in food, nutrition, physiology, behavior changes, and more. He or she will assess your current diet, food preferences, diet and health goals, medical history, medications, laboratory tests, and the results from your home blood glucose monitoring. Since you are not the same as your neighbor or friend with diabetes, and your diabetes is not the same as your friend's or neighbor's, your diet plan will also be different. Do not expect a diabetic diet from a tear pad when you visit with a registered dietitian. You will walk out of the office with a solid meal plan tailored just to you.

Fear: I'll never be able to eat my favorite foods again.
Reality: A registered dietitian will show you how to fit your favorite foods into your meal plan.

Fear: The dietitian will tell me to eat kale and tofu and other foods I hate.
Reality: The dietitian will tailor the meal plan to your food preferences, but encourage you to try new foods.

Fear: I'll never be able to follow a healthy diet plan.
Reality: Your dietitian will help you make the appropriate changes at a pace that suits you. Together you will set achievable goals that will bring about the results you seek. Then you'll set more goals and more goals. Your registered dietitian nutritionist is your partner and your coach.

Fear: A visit to a dietitian will be a waste of time and money because I can learn about a diabetic diet on the web and in magazines.
Reality: The quality of diet advice on the Internet and in the media is questionable. While some is spot on, most of it is inaccurate or incomplete and written by people without medical training. Worse, a lot of it is purposefully misleading to get you to buy a diet product. A registered dietitian nutritionist is professionally trained and will provide you with personalized advice.

Make the Most of Your Visit

Learn about insurance coverage. Many insurance companies, including Medicare, now cover medical nutrition therapy for diabetes management as well as many other diagnoses and health concerns. Call your insurance company to find out what your policy covers and how many visits you may have with the registered dietitian nutritionist. Your health-care provider's office or the dietitian's office may also be able to help you with this.

Gather things for your visit. The dietitian will likely want a list of your medications and supplements and your recent lab work. You can bring these or ask someone at your health-care provider's office to send them.

Additionally, bring your blood glucose log, a list of any questions you have, food labels from foods you eat often, and menus from your favorite restaurants.

Decide if you should go alone. If someone else does the cooking and shopping, it's wise to bring that person along. Even if you do those chores, feel free to bring the person who offers you support. If you feel that it's easier to be open and that you'll be more comfortable if you go alone, that's what you should do.

Be honest. The dietitian is there to help you, not to judge you. If you skip breakfast, binge on ice cream, get up in the middle of the night to eat cookies, don't know how to cook, drink too much, or recently gained a lot of weight, share this information. Otherwise, your plan will not truly be personalized. If the dietitian offers suggestions you don't like, say so and say why.

Be open-minded. You will not be forced to do anything you don't want to do, but it is smart to carefully consider the dietitian's suggestions. Avoid knee-jerk negative reactions about advice to eat breakfast, monitor blood glucose more often, add vegetables to your meals, or anything that you think you don't want to do. Talk it out. You may find that you can do part of it or that you can put that goal aside until another day.

Set specific goals with your dietitian. It's not enough to simply learn new information. To make good progress, you must have a plan with specific strategies. As you saw in chapter 13, your goals should be so specific that you know exactly how to proceed. For example, will you consume a set amount of carbohydrates at each of your meals and snacks? Will you eat a piece of fruit at lunch every day, or will you pack lunch at least twice weekly? These are the types of goals that set you down a clear path to success.

Schedule your next appointment. Nearly everyone will benefit from additional appointments. Among other things, follow-up visits give you the opportunity to discuss your progress, ask questions, revise your goals and set new ones, get additional support and encouragement, and discuss strategies for vacations, holidays, sick days, and more. Ask the dietitian what to do should you have questions between appointments. Some dietitians prefer to talk by phone; others like to use email.

Physical Activity Support and Advice

If you have no health problems that limit your choices of physical activity, your nurse, registered dietitian, or other certified diabetes educator likely can help you get started. However, if you have complications, if your fitness level is poor, if you have goals of an athlete, or if you want to increase the pace of your progress, you will benefit from the help of a fitness expert. Ask your health-care provider if you should see an exercise physiologist or other expert. Ask if there are local wellness programs for people with diabetes.

If you have the okay to exercise, but need or want additional guidance, seek out a certified personal trainer who can help you create a customized fitness program. You can find personal trainers at gyms, fitness studios, recreation centers, and online or in the phone book. Some will even come to your home. Ask friends and health professionals for recommendations. Use the following checklist to help you find the right trainer. This trainer is ...

- ✓ certified by a nationally recognized and accredited organization such as the American College of Sports Medicine (ACSM), American Council on Exercise (ACE), Cooper Institute, National Academy of Sports Medicine (NASM), National Council on Strength and Fitness (NCSF), National Exercise Trainers Association (NETA), National Federation of Professional Trainers (NFPT), and National Strength and Conditioning Association (NSCA)

- ✓ recommended by someone you know and trust

- ✓ trained to perform cardiopulmonary resuscitation (CPR)

- ✓ experienced in working with people your age and with your health conditions

- ✓ carrying liability insurance

- ✓ flexible to your schedule

- ✓ affordable

- ✓ personable and likable

Just like a registered dietitian, your certified personal trainer should be able to tailor your program to your health needs and your preferences. You should have specific goals to get started and to improve your fitness level. A personal trainer should be with you when you work out and give you exercises to perform on your own if you are able.

Take Action

Ask for referrals to nutrition and fitness professionals if you need more guidance.

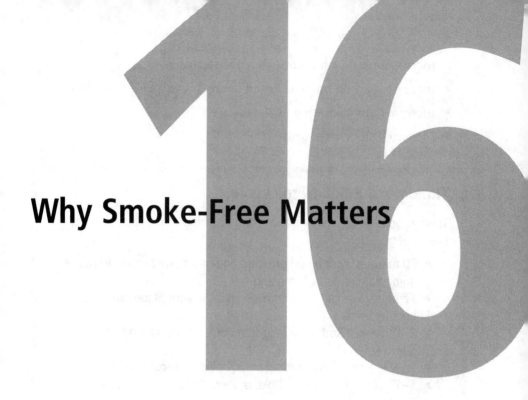

Why Smoke-Free Matters

The combination of diabetes and smoking is even more harmful than either alone. The combination puts you at great risk of developing heart disease. Even minimal smoking increases the risk of developing heart disease, but the more you smoke, the greater is your risk. Smoking also increases the risk for stroke, peripheral arterial disease, and aortic aneurysm. People with diabetes who smoke are also more likely to develop the microvascular complications of diabetes—such as nerve and eye diseases—earlier than if they did not smoke. Smoking also increases the risk of health problems that are unrelated to blood vessels, such as cancer and hip fractures.

Smoking cigars and pipes also increases the risk of premature death. Even being near someone who is smoking can be harmful. The American Heart Association estimates that secondhand smoke causes 22,700–69,600 premature deaths yearly from heart and blood vessel diseases.

How Smoking Damages the Heart and Blood Vessels

Smoking damages blood cells, blood vessels, and the heart in many ways:

> Damages the blood vessel lining causing endothelial dysfunction

> Decreases HDL cholesterol

- Increases modification of LDL cholesterol
- Increases carbon monoxide and decreases oxygen in the blood
- Increases blood clotting
- Increases blood pressure

Timeline of Smoke-Free Living

There is good news even with smoking: Quitting can reverse some of the damage. After:

- 20 minutes: Your blood pressure and heart rate recover from the immediate effects of smoking.
- 12 hours: The carbon monoxide levels in your blood return to healthy levels.
- 2–12 weeks: Both your lung function and circulation begin to improve.
- 1 year: Your risk for coronary heart disease is cut in half.
- 5–15 years: Your risk of stoke is about the same as that of a non-smoker.
- 10 years: Your lung cancer death rate approaches half of what it would be if you continued to smoke. Your risk of developing other cancers also decreases.

Source: American Heart Association

Becoming Smoke-Free

Quitting smoking is very hard. If you've tried before, you already know that. The nicotine in smoke is addictive. It quickly reaches your brain, where it can temporarily relieve stress and enhance mood. In fact, nicotine from cigarette smoke reaches the brain faster than drugs that are given intravenously (through an IV). Once the effects wear off, it leaves the smoker craving more. Withdrawal symptoms include anxiety, irritability, depression, poor concentration, sleep problems, headaches, and more. Some smokers quit on their own. Others need help to break the addiction or to break the behavioral habits associated with smoking.

Changing behaviors. Your environment influences your desires. If you attend a staff meeting where there are trays of sweets, for example, you may want to eat a donut. Try to identify your smoking triggers. Do you typically take smoke breaks with coworkers or smoke every morning with a cup of coffee? Once you identify your triggers, plan to change them. For example, take a break with coworkers who don't smoke, or drink iced tea instead of hot coffee. Many people find chewing sugarless gum or holding and sucking on cinnamon sticks (sticks of real cinnamon, not candy) helpful. It's a good idea to ask your friends and family for support; spend time with nonsmokers and ex-smokers; remove all cigarettes from your home, car, and place of work; write and review your list of reasons to quit smoking; practice stress management; and get to bed on time.

Breaking addiction. Nicotine replacement therapy (NRT) helps smokers wean themselves from nicotine. It comes in the form of gum, patches, inhalers, nasal sprays, and lozenges. Some require prescriptions. Use NRT for just a few weeks or months as instructed. To be successful, you must taper the dose before you completely stop using NRT. There are other prescription drugs that can help you as well. Your health-care provider may want you to take one of them with NRT or by itself.

You may see other products for sale with promises to make you nicotine- or cigarette-free. One such product is a nicotine lollipop. The U.S. Food and Drug Administration does not allow the sale of this product. The electronic cigarette (e-cigarette) is another product that may catch your interest. However, it was neither designed as an aid to quit smoking nor approved as one. The e-cigarette was developed to allow smokers a way of getting nicotine in places where smoking is not permitted. It comes with cartridges of nicotine and flavorings. Researchers have not yet determined the safety of e-cigarettes or their usefulness in helping smokers quit, though at least one study shows e-cigarettes to be as effective as the nicotine patch.

Structured support. There are support programs available online, by telephone, and in your community. Look into the following resources. The American Cancer Society suggests choosing a program that lasts at least 2 weeks and has a minimum of four sessions for at least 15 minutes each.

> ➤ American Cancer Society: 1-800-227-2345, cancer.org

> ➤ American Heart Association: 1-800-242-8721, heart.org

> ➤ National Cancer Institute: 1-877-448-7848, smokefree.gov

> ➤ National Association of Tobacco Cessation Quitlines: 1-800-784-8669, naquitline.org

Pick a quit date. The American Cancer Society recommends picking a date to become smoke-free. This allows you time to prepare to be successful. Your quit date, however, should not be so far away that you lose interest in quitting and change your mind. You will need a plan that includes whether or not to use NRT or prescription drugs and whether or not you'll attend support meetings. If you plan to take prescription medications, you may need to start them a week or two before giving up tobacco.

You will also need to prepare your environment. Stock up on sugarless gum and cinnamon sticks if you plan to use them. Get rid of your ashtrays and lighters. Talk to your friends and coworkers about your plan and how they can help you. Gather reading materials from the American Cancer Society, the American Heart Association, or a similar organization. Finally, if you have tried to quit smoking before, reflect on those past attempts to see what derailed you and how you can avoid those situations again.

Choose Your Support Program Wisely

The American Cancer Society warns against programs that:

➤ promise instant success
➤ claim that quitting is easy
➤ use shots, pills, or secret ingredients
➤ claim 100% success rate
➤ charge a very high fee
➤ fail to provide references and phone numbers of previous program users or attendees

Take Action

If you smoke or use any form of tobacco, pick a date to quit. Ask your family, friends, and health-care provider for support.

Understanding Glucose-Lowering Medications

People with diabetes frequently take one or more medications to control blood glucose, as well as medications for blood pressure and blood lipids, if necessary. See chapters 7 and 9 for a discussion of blood pressure and lipids medications. If you have type 1 diabetes, you require insulin either by injection or through an insulin pump. Most people with type 1 diabetes, if not using a pump, will take three or more injections per day. Some people with type 2 diabetes do not take any medications, but most do. In fact, research suggests that starting medication early in the treatment of type 2 diabetes is associated with improved long-term health outcomes. It's not uncommon for people with type 2 diabetes to take multiple medications for optimal blood glucose control. This is not a sign of failure. Type 2 diabetes is a progressive disease, meaning that over time, it becomes more difficult to manage blood glucose levels. Many people with type 2 diabetes will eventually need to take insulin as well, but again, this does not mean that the individual has done something wrong.

Taking your medications as prescribed to keep your blood glucose level under control is critical for your overall well-being. As you saw in chapter 1, diabetes is linked to endothelial dysfunction and atherosclerosis. Additionally, good blood glucose control can prevent or delay diabetic complications including eye, nerve, and kidney diseases. The table below summarizes the actions of common diabetes medications.

Glucose-Lowering Medications

Type of Drug	Common Name	Actions	Heart-Related Effects
Biguanide (pill)	Metformin (Glucophage)	Reduces the amount of glucose released by the liver and decreases insulin resistance by muscle cells.	Facilitates weight loss and improves HDL cholesterol, LDL cholesterol, and triglycerides.
Sulfonylureas (pill)	Glimepiride (Amaryl) Glipizide (Glucotrol) Glyburide (Diabeta, Micronase, Glynase)	Stimulates the beta-cells of the pancreas to increase insulin production.	May make weight control more difficult.
Meglitinides (pill)	Repaglinide (Prandin) Nateglinide (Starlix)	Stimulates the beta-cells of the pancreas to increase insulin production. They are faster-acting and work for a shorter amount of time than sulfonylureas.	May make weight control slightly more difficult.
Thiazolidine-diones Also called glitazones or TZDs (pill)	Pioglitizone (Actos) Rosiglitazone (Avandia)	Increases insulin sensitivity of the liver, muscle, and fat tissues.	May cause fluid retention, edema, and weight gain. May improve blood cholesterol and triglyceride levels.
Alpha-glucosidase inhibitors (pill)	Acarbose (Precose) Miglitol (Glycet)	Slows digestion and absorption of carbohydrate.	May slightly lower LDL and triglyceride levels.

*Not a complete list

Type of Drug	Common Name	Actions	Heart-Related Effects
Dipeptidyl peptidase IV inhibitors Also called DPP-4 inhibitors (pill)	Sitagliptin (Januvia) Saxagliptin (Onglyza) Linagliptin (Tradjenta) Alogliptin (Nesina)	Increases the amount of incretin hormones, thus increasing insulin production and decreasing glucose release from the liver.	May decrease blood triglyceride levels.
Sodium-glucose co-transporter 2 inhibitors Also called SGLT2 inhibitors (pill)	Canagliflozin (Invokana) Dapagliflozin (Farxiga)	Reduces glucose in the blood by causing more than usual amounts to be excreted in the urine.	May slightly lower weight and blood pressure. May increase LDL cholesterol.
Incretin mimetic (injectable)	Exenatide (Byetta) Liraglitude (Victoza) Exenatide extended release (Bydureon)	Mimics the effect of incretin hormones to increase insulin production and decrease glucagon production.	Facilitates weight loss by reducing appetite. May improve triglyceride levels in the blood.
Amylin analogue (injectable, used in conjunction with mealtime insulin in type 1 or type 2 diabetes)	Pramlintide (Symlin)	Slows digestion, which delays glucose from entering the bloodstream. Also decreases glucose released by the liver by suppressing the hormone glucagon.	Facilitates weight loss by decreasing appetite and by slowing the passage of food from the stomach.

*Not a complete list

Type of Drug	Common Name	Actions	Heart-Related Effects
Insulin (inject-able, required in all people with type 1 diabetes, also used in type 2 diabetes)	Long-acting insulin: Glargine (Lantus) Detemir (Levemir) Intermediate-acting insulin: NPH (Humulin N, Novolin N, Relion N) Short-acting insulin: Regular (Humulin R, Novolin R, Relion R) Rapid-acting insulin: Lispro (Humalog) Aspart (NovoLog) Glulisine (Apidra)	Replaces the body's natural insulin in type 1 diabetes and is used as an adjunct therapy in type 2 diabetes when the natural insulin is insufficient. Increases the passage of glucose from the bloodstream into the cells and decreases the production of glucose by the liver.	Often makes weight control more difficult.

*Not a complete list

Source: *Medical Management of Type 2 Diabetes*, 7th edition, American Diabetes Association (2012)

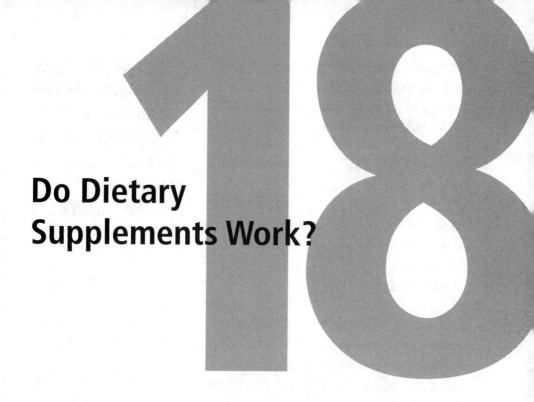

Do Dietary Supplements Work?

Walking down the supplement aisle of your local pharmacy can be quite overwhelming. There are pills, powders, liquids, capsules, herbs, vitamins, and minerals. Supplements may be sold individually or in combination. Some are marketed specifically to people with diabetes.

Helpful or harmful? Both. Some supplements are useful, but others are downright dangerous. Still others are somewhere in the middle. The bottom line when considering taking supplements is to educate yourself, proceed with caution, and discuss their use with your health-care provider.

Buyer Beware

The words *natural* and *dietary supplements* sound harmless. What could be bad about something that is natural and supplements your diet? Just because something is natural doesn't mean it is safe. Tobacco, after all, is natural, but it is known to be unsafe. Some supplements interact with medications and have side effects. For example, fenugreek may cause excessive bleeding during surgery, and ginseng may increase blood pressure and interfere with the blood-thinning medication warfarin.

Additionally, what's on the label may not be what's in the bottle.

Dietary supplements do not have the same level of oversight that medications have. Sometimes the supplement contains a different dose than the amount listed on the label. Supplements may even be contaminated with other herbs, pesticides, lead and other metals, and even prescription drugs. In one study of supplement contents, only 52% of echinacea products were accurately labeled, and 10% of them contained no echinacea at all.

No federal agency evaluates whether or not supplements actually do what they claim, if the labeling is accurate, or if the product is contaminated.

Regulation of Dietary Supplements. Under the 1994 Dietary Supplement Health and Education Act, the U.S. Food and Drug Administration (FDA) has limited oversight over dietary supplements. The manufacturer does not need to provide the FDA with data that shows the supplement to be safe or effective. In fact, the FDA would need to prove that the product was unsafe before taking it off the market. In contrast, drug manufacturers must provide data proving both safety and effectiveness before putting a drug on the market. For this reason, it is a poor assumption that it is better or safer to take supplements instead of medications.

Manufacturers are not allowed to claim that the supplement treats, prevents, or cures an illness. They may, however, make claims such as these:

Maintains cell integrity.
Provides 100% of the RDA for vitamin C.
Maintains a healthy liver.
Supports normal blood glucose.
Helps maintain a healthy circulatory system.

Keep in mind that manufacturers do not need to give evidence to the FDA regarding statements about the effectiveness of supplements, but the label must state the following: "This statement has not been evaluated by the Food and Drug Administration (FDA). This product is not intended to diagnose, treat, cure, or prevent any disease."

Finding Reliable Information about Dietary Supplements

You may be wondering if there is any accurate information about dietary supplements available. Since regulations are lax, you will need to do your homework. There are several agencies and organizations that offer guidance. Start with one or more of these and discuss supplement use with your health-care provider.

National Institutes of Health: Office of Dietary Supplements (ods.od.nih. gov): Learn about regulations; get fact sheets for vitamins, minerals, and herbal supplements; download a free app.

National Institutes of Health and U.S. National Library of Medicine: Dietary Supplements Label Database (dsld.nlm.nih.gov/dsld): Compare labels from various supplement products.

National Institutes of Health: National Center for Complementary and Alternative Medicine (nccam.nih.gov): Find tips on being an informed consumer; get fact sheets on various herbs; learn the newest research about certain supplements.

Natural Medicines Comprehensive Database (naturaldatabase. therapeuticresearch.com): Search for a supplement to learn about safety, effectiveness, mechanism of action, side effects, interactions with food and drugs, and more. There is a fee to access this database.

Consumer Lab (consumerlab.com): Search for a supplement to learn about the purity of various brands. There is a fee to access this site.

The American Diabetes Association Guide to Herbs and Nutritional Supplements by Laura Shane McWhorter: Reviews more than three dozen supplements of interest to people with diabetes; covers uses, dose, scientific evidence, side effects, and drug interactions.

Choosing a Supplement

If you've done your research and spoken with your health-care provider, use these guidelines to pick a suitable product.

➤ Look for a seal of approval from one of the following independent testing organizations.

▷ U.S. Pharmacopeia (USP) Dietary Supplement Verification (usp. org): Indicates that the product is pure, it will dissolve properly, the ingredients are labeled accurately, and the manufacturer uses good manufacturing practices.

▷ NSF International (nsf.org): Indicates that the product is pure and accurately labeled and that the manufacturer uses good manufacturing practices.

> ▷ Consumer Lab (consumerlab.com): Indicates that the ingredients are labeled accurately and free of contaminants.

- ➤ Purchase a brand only if the label clearly indicates a way to reach the company should you have questions.

- ➤ Avoid products that claim to have no side effects or claim that the product is a "breakthrough."

- ➤ Do not take any supplement that claims to cure a disease.

- ➤ Avoid mixtures of supplements. Products with many ingredients are more likely to have harmful effects, and it is more difficult to learn which ingredient is helping or hurting. A general multivitamin mineral supplement is the exception to this guideline.

- ➤ Do not take more than the recommended dosage.

Talk to Your Health-Care Provider

Get answers to your health-care questions from health-care providers, not from salespeople in health food or supplement stores. Talk to your health-care provider, pharmacist, registered dietitian nutritionist, or certified diabetes educator. Share a list of your medications *and* dietary supplements with your health-care providers. Include the dosages of both medications and supplements. Ask your health-care provider how the supplement may affect your blood glucose, blood pressure, and other health conditions. Ask about side effects and what to do if you are scheduled for surgery. Even if your health-care provider discourages their use, you must be honest and forthcoming about your use of supplements, because your health-care provider may attribute a side effect of the supplement to a drug or prescribe an additional drug that may interact with a supplement.

Take Action

Add any supplements that you take to your list of medications. Talk to your health-care provider about all of your supplements.

Supplements in Action

Maura has had type 2 diabetes for more than 6 years and has managed it with medications, diet, and exercise. Her A1C has fluctuated between 6.6% and 7.2%. Recently, despite an increased effort with diet and exercise, Maura's A1C rose to 7.8%. She had read that cinnamon is good for blood glucose control. Since she loves cinnamon anyway, she started adding it to her foods at most meals. She added it to coffee, oatmeal, cottage cheese, sweet potatoes, even salads, stews, chicken, and beef. Several months later, Maura's A1C dropped to 7.4%. It's hard to know if the cinnamon helped to lower her A1C, but it's possible. Maura had no side effects.

Maura shared her story with her brother Jake, who has had type 2 diabetes for 10 years. He thought he'd give cinnamon a try, but since he doesn't like the flavor, he decided to take cinnamon capsules. He visited a few websites listed above and learned that *Cinnamomum cassia*, also called Chinese cinnamon, is the form studied for use in diabetes and that the doses in the studies range from 1 to 6 grams daily. He found a cinnamon supplement made from the suggested variety of cinnamon in 1-gram capsules. The bottle was labeled with ingredient and dosage information and the manufacturer's phone number and website. It had a quality seal from one of the independent testing organizations listed above. Jake bought a bottle of 200 capsules. The next morning, when he was counting out his pills for the day, he hesitated when he came to the cinnamon bottle. He wondered how it might interact with his prescription medications. Good thing Jake decided to call the pharmacist. She advised Jake not to take the cinnamon supplement because it could interfere with his blood-thinning medications.

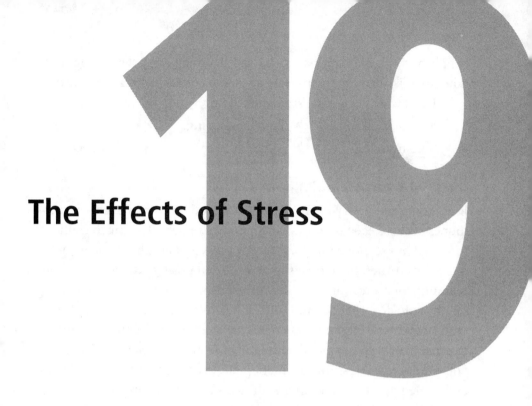

The Effects of Stress

Physical stress, like a broken leg, the flu, or surgery, often increases blood glucose in people with diabetes. In fact, researchers have even found that sleep deprivation worsens insulin resistance, making blood glucose levels more difficult to manage.

The effects of emotional stress are not so clear. A number of physiological changes occur when stress hormones are activated, and some people find that controlling their blood glucose becomes more difficult. Yet others report no changes in their level of control. While it's not been proven that emotional stress causes heart disease or diabetes or that it even raises the risk for either disease, we do know that it can indirectly affect our health by distracting us from our everyday self-care efforts.

How Does Stress Affect You?

People react to stress in various ways. Even the same person may react one way today, but a different way next week or next month. Sometimes people become so busy or so distracted that they don't even recognize how stress is affecting them. Here are some common stress responses.

- Headache
- Stomachache
- Sore muscles
- Clenched jaw
- Trouble sleeping
- Anger
- Sadness
- Anxiety
- Impatience

Develop a Stress Management Plan

Diabetes or not, everyone needs to learn good stress management techniques because each of us deals with daily stressors. Too much traffic, too much noise, not enough money or time, anxiety about a new job or a sick family member—the list goes on. Even positive stressors, such as planning for a vacation, a holiday celebration, or a new baby, can bring on physiological changes and spur unhealthful behaviors. If you deal with stress by eating, smoking, drinking alcohol, or sleeping too little or too much, or if you respond by treating yourself or others badly, then you need a new stress management plan. Use the following techniques and strategies for both dealing with stress and preventing it.

Breathe deeply. Take a few deep breaths to relax your body and clear your mind.

Hit the hay. A good night's sleep makes it so much easier to deal with everyday annoyances like aggressive drivers and an onslaught of telemarketers, as well as bigger problems like a difficult job. An occasional good night, however, is not enough. You need sound sleep for 7 or 8 hours nightly. If you have trouble getting to bed on time or falling asleep, start a bedtime ritual to prepare yourself for sleep. This might be a routine of washing your face, reading a few pages in a good book, and sipping a cup of decaf tea. Choose any soothing activities that help you relax. If you need more help, seek the advice of a member of your health-care team.

Exercise. Being physically active is good for your stress level and good to help you sleep soundly. Even if you only have a few minutes daily, use them to be physically active.

Take control. If having too many responsibilities at work is your source of stress, a conversation with your coworkers or boss may lead you to a solution. If your worries come from learning that your blood glucose or cholesterol levels are elevated, reining in out-of-control food portions is a good first step. Use food records, blood glucose records, and more frequent blood glucose monitoring to put you in control.

Sometimes you really don't have control over the source of stress. For example, you may be worried about a family member's health. If you have already sought out good medical care and have learned what you can about the illness, there may be nothing more that you can do to change the outcome. But you can still feel empowered and deal better with stress by controlling those aspects of your life that you can influence. Get to bed on time, pack a healthful lunch, spend time with people who make you happy, volunteer for an important cause, participate in daily physical activity, and engage in other self-care behaviors.

Seek help. Help comes in many ways. Perhaps a family member can wash the dinner dishes so you can take a walk. If your diabetes is out of control, make an appointment with your diabetes educator, registered dietitian nutritionist, or health-care provider. Maybe confiding in a friend is what you need. If stress is affecting your work, family life, or happiness, you may need additional help from a psychotherapist. Ask for a referral.

Be a joiner. Join a support group for people with diabetes or heart disease. Ask a health professional to recommend one to you, or call a local hospital to see if they facilitate support groups. Additionally, you can visit the websites of the American Diabetes Association, American Heart Association, and the American Stroke Association to look for a group in your area or for an online support group. Message boards are another way to connect. Visit diabetes.org/messageboards to join, or simply lurk on the ADA message board. On Twitter, follow the hashtag #DSMA (diabetes social media advocacy) to join conversations about all things affecting people with diabetes.

Stay positive. There are many other things you can do to stay positive. Cuddle a pet, spend a few minutes in prayer or meditation, keep a daily gratitude journal, have a good belly laugh, speak nicely to yourself and others, volunteer, start a new hobby or revisit an old one, listen to music. This list is endless, but in sum, it's a list of things that nurture you, relax you, and feed your soul.

Take Action

Identify suitable methods to control stress and practice them daily.

You Can Prevent Long-Term Complications

As you learned in earlier chapters, controlling the ABCs of diabetes care will go far in helping you prevent heart disease and stroke. These complications are known as macrovascular or large blood vessel diseases. The same efforts will also help you prevent microvascular or small blood vessel problems. This chapter introduces the microvascular complications of diabetes.

Though A1C goals should always be individualized, maintaining an A1C of about 7% or below has been shown to reduce the microvascular complications of diabetes. Additionally, you should visit with your health-care team regularly to screen for complications and other health problems. See the recommended health maintenance schedule at the end of this chapter.

Retinopathy: Eye Disease

Retinopathy is a disease of the eye's retina, the region of the eye that senses light. In nonproliferative retinopathy, the small blood vessels in the back of the eye swell and weaken. They can leak blood, fluid, and fats into the eye. This type of retinopathy can progress to proliferative retinopathy, in which new blood vessels form in the retina. Unfortunately, they are weak and rupture easily, causing scar tissue and blocking vision. An ophthalmologist (an eye specialist) performs a dilated retinal eye exam to screen for and monitor retinopathy.

➤ Report visual problems immediately to get sight-saving care. You may get blurry vision if your blood glucose is quite elevated. This usually disappears when glucose is better controlled.

➤ High blood glucose and high blood pressure both increase the risk of developing retinopathy.

Nephropathy: Kidney Disease

A healthy kidney has millions of tiny blood vessels, called capillaries, that filter blood. They remove toxins and waste materials and excrete them through the urine. A healthy kidney will leave proteins and other nutrients in the blood. If these blood vessels are damaged, they may leave toxins to build up in the blood and allow proteins and other important compounds to be lost through the urine. The condition in which a small amount of protein leaks into the urine is called microalbuminuria. This can progress to macroalbuminuria, the condition in which large amounts of protein go into your urine. Your health-care provider will screen for and monitor kidney problems by measuring protein in your urine.

➤ Both high blood glucose and high blood pressure increase the risk of developing nephropathy.

➤ Kidney damage can also cause high blood pressure, which accelerates the disease even more.

➤ Treating high blood pressure with medications, weight loss, and dietary measures will help prevent or slow the progression of diabetic kidney disease.

Neuropathy: Nerve Damage

The nervous system affects many parts of your body. It tells your muscles when to contract; it affects how food moves through your digestive tract and how urine flows; it even affects your heart rate, blood pressure, and more. About half of all people with diabetes have some sort of nerve damage. Peripheral neuropathy is the most common type. It causes tingling, numbness, burning, or other pain in the feet, legs, hands, or arms. Autonomic neuropathy affects the nerves that control the bladder, sexual organs, digestive system, sweat glands, circulatory system, and more. Among other things, neuropathy may cause foot pain, slow passage of food from the stomach, cause an abnormal heart rate, make it difficult or impossible to recognize hypoglycemia, and result in an inadequate sexual response. Your health-care provider should perform a comprehensive foot exam each year, measure your blood pressure, and listen to your heart at each medical visit, as well as discuss any abnormalities or health concerns.

➤ Often symptoms of neuropathy improve when blood glucose becomes better controlled. Medications can also help manage symptoms.

➤ Check your feet daily for the presence of sores, calluses, and blisters. Use a mirror, if necessary, or ask a family member to help you.

Additional Problems

Dental problems are frequently more severe among people with diabetes than among the general population. Hearing loss is more common in people with diabetes. Additionally, high blood glucose and problems with sweat glands can cause the skin to become dry and itchy, which may lead to sores and infections.

Diabetes Health Maintenance Schedule

What to Do	When to Do It	American Diabetes Association Targets for Many People with Diabetes*
Check A1C	Every 6 months	<7%
	Every 3 months if you're not meeting goals or your treatment plan changes	
Review blood glucose monitoring records	Every routine visit	70–130 mg/dl before meals
		<180 mg/dl 1–2 hours after the start of the meal

*All targets should be individualized. Discuss your goals with your health-care provider.

What to Do	When to Do It	American Diabetes Association Targets for Many People with Diabetes*
Measure blood pressure	Every routine visit	<140/80 mmHg for those with diabetes and hypertension (Anyone with blood pressure that is >120/80 mmHg should initiate lifestyle changes to improve their numbers.)
Get lipid panel (cholesterol & triglycerides)	Every year typically Every 2 years if your health-care provider deems you to be at low risk	LDL: <100 mg/dl LDL: <70 mg/dl for individuals with CVD HDL: >40 mg/dl in men >50 mg/dl in women Triglycerides: <150 mg/dl
Test urine protein (indicates the health of your kidneys)	Every year if you have type 2 diabetes Every year once you have had type 1 diabetes for at least 5 years	<30 µg/mg creatinine
Test blood creatinine (indicates the health of your kidneys)	Every year	Varies according to age, gender and race
Have comprehensive eye exam	Shortly after the diagnosis of type 2 diabetes and every 1–2 years thereafter Within 5 years of diagnosis of type 1 diabetes and every 1–2 years thereafter	Normal, healthy eyes
Have comprehensive foot exam to include inspection, assessment of foot pulses and loss of sensation (Check your own feet daily)	Every year	Normal, no loss of sensation, healthy circulation
Have dental exam & cleaning	Every 6 months	Healthy teeth and gums
Get flu vaccine	Every year in the fall	—

*All targets should be individualized. Discuss your goals with your health-care provider.

What to Do	When to Do It	American Diabetes Association Targets for Many People with Diabetes*
Get pneumonia vaccine	Once in your life if you are over age 65 If you get the shot before you are 65, you may need another .	—
Receive diabetes education and/or medical nutrition therapy	At diagnosis and each year after	—
Measure weight	Every routine visit	Varies

*All targets should be individualized. Discuss your goals with your health-care provider.

Take Action

Keep track of your screening results and when your next screening should occur. Discuss each test with your health-care provider. Examine your feet daily. Learn more about caring for your feet and preventing other complications at diabetes.org.

Finding Reliable Information

Whether you are looking for information about diabetes, heart disease, or any other health concern, there is no shortage of information. Unfortunately, much of it is incorrect, and even worse, some is downright fraudulent. Seeking information and advice from reputable sources is critical.

Because there is no one exactly like you with your medical history, daily activities, food preferences, and health goals, it's reasonable that your diabetes management plan should be individualized. Information from a friend or family member may be helpful, or it may not even apply to you. This is where your health-care team comes in. It's smart to verify new information with a medical professional. Your physician or other primary-care provider looks at your unique health profile when prescribing medications and making other recommendations. A registered dietitian nutritionist helps you plan meals that fit your budget, time constraints, preferences, cooking abilities, and medical conditions. Certified diabetes educators (CDEs) help you make the most of your blood glucose results. They make sense of that information and offer suggestions for changes in your exercise routine or diet. They may work with your health-care provider to change medications if necessary. Diabetes educators help interpret your lab results and teach you to care for your feet and be on the lookout for the complications of diabetes, including heart disease. Each of these health professionals can help you sort through contradictory medical advice and make sense of the health claims you see on the Internet, in magazines, and on supplement and food labels.

Get Educated

If you haven't already attended a diabetes education program, ask your health-care provider for a referral. Diabetes education programs, often called diabetes self-management education (DSME) programs, are usually run by diabetes educators who are nurses and dietitians. Some programs have pharmacists, behavioral counselors, exercise specialists, and other experts, too. These classes may run for several days or weeks and often total 9 or 10 hours. You will learn about the disease process; managing blood glucose, blood pressure, and blood cholesterol; meal planning; self-monitoring blood glucose; medications; signs and symptoms of high blood glucose and low blood glucose; participating in physical activity; and more. Before signing up for a diabetes education program, ask if it is recognized by either the American Diabetes Association or accredited by the American Association of Diabetes Educators. Then call your insurance company to find out if they will pay for all or part of the program.

Reputable Resources

American Diabetes Association: diabetes.org
> *Find information about caring for and preventing diabetes.*

Academy of Nutrition and Dietetics: eatright.org
> *Find information about healthy eating and locate a registered dietitian nutritionist in your area.*

American Association of Diabetes Educators: diabeteseducator.org
> *Locate a certified diabetes educator in your area.*

American Heart Association: heart.org
> *Find information about preventing and treating heart disease.*

American Stroke Association: strokeassociation.org
Learn about preventing and treating stroke.

Centers for Disease Control and Prevention: cdc.gov/diabetes
Find statistics and general information about diabetes.

Juvenile Diabetes Research Foundation: jdrf.org
Get information about living with and managing type 1 diabetes.

National Cholesterol Education Program of the National Heart, Lung, and Blood Institute: nhlbi.nih.gov/about/ncep
Get fact sheets and brochures about cholesterol and management of high blood cholesterol.

National Diabetes Education Program: ndep.nih.gov
Find handouts and fact sheets about preventing diabetes.

National Institute of Diabetes and Digestive and Kidney Diseases of the National Institutes of Health: niddk.nih.gov
Find basic information about meal planning, insulin, diabetes and pregnancy, and more.

Books

Both the American Diabetes Association and the American Heart Association publish books and cookbooks that will help you manage or prevent diabetes and heart disease. You can find them at diabetes.org, heart.org, and online and in traditional bookstores.

Take Action

Empower yourself by finding the answers to all of your questions. Start with your health-care team and the resources listed above.